While the author of this book has made every effort to ensure that the information contained is as accurate and up-to-date as possible at the time of publication, medical and pharmaceutical knowledge is constantly changing and the application of it to particular circumstances depends on many factors. This book should not be used as an alternative to specialist medical advice and it is recommended that readers always consult a qualified medical professional for individual advice before following any new diet or health programme. The author and the publishers cannot be held responsible for any errors and omissions that can be found in the text, or any actions that may be taken by a reader as a result of any reliance on the information contained in the text, which are taken entirely at the reader's own risk.

Super Blend Me!
ISBN: 978-0-9547664-9-8

First published in 2017 by Juice Master Publications.
Copyright © Jason Vale & Juice Master Publications 2017.

Jason Vale has asserted his right to be identified as the author of this publication in accordance with the Copyright, Designs and Patents Act 1988.

'Juice Master', 'Juice Master Publications' and the 'Juicy Man' logo are trademarks of The Juice Master Limited, registered in England #04632887.
www.juicemaster.com

Brands and product names are acknowledged as trademarks of their respective owners.

Written by Jason Vale with acknowledged contributions.
Photography by Lightmill.

JASON VALE
SUPER BLEND ME!

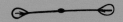

"I have actually got into my size 8 jeans
with a little room around my belly for
the 1st time since having a baby!!"
JOANNE

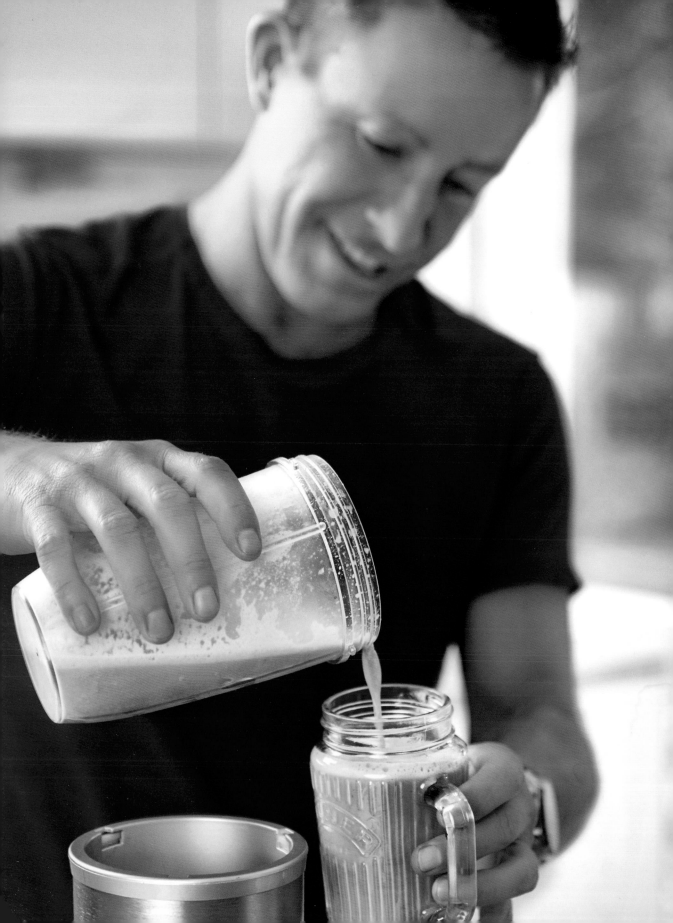

CONTENTS

A
BIG
High Five!

I'd like to say a big high five to the key players who helped to make this book possible...

My Katie, my rock, recipe creator, ideas factory, truly amazing human and all round love of my life!

Alex Leith, photographer extraordinaire, design king, and all round VERY good egg!

Andrea Wells, my wonderful PA, life organiser and all round VERY top banana!

Oliver Saunders, design wizard and all round good avocado! (*I've already used egg, and I guess avocado is just as arbitrary, so why not!*)

Me, well, seeing as I did write the thing! :)

The Whole Juicy Team! Although I've thanked the main players in the creation of this book, the *whole* juicy team ultimately helped to make it happen, even if they didn't realise it. We are blessed to have incredible, genuinely lovely people working with us, who love the fact that we are in the business of helping to make a difference. Whether it's the lovely Skye and Alison over at Juice Master Delivered, making sure the quality of all our juice / blend plans and the level of service remains the highest in the industry; Marcus, Oliver, Dan, Alex and Chris over at Juicy HQ, our tech wizards who keep all of the cogs well-oiled and moving; the lovely retreats booking team, Nina, Joanna and Meriam; or Mairi, who takes care of all things Juice Master Academy e-learning. They all play a huge part in what we do. Then we have the truly amazing retreats team (of which there are far too many to mention, but you know who you are!). Cary, Chris and Elliot from our fulfilment house, who ensure the safe and swift delivery of all your juicing / blending goodies and of course Daska and Matt, who produce our wonderful *Juiced! Magazine*.

There are no doubt many more who I have missed, but it takes a full and committed team to make all of this possible and to allow me the freedom to write and be creative – so thank you and a massive **HIGH FIVE** to you all!

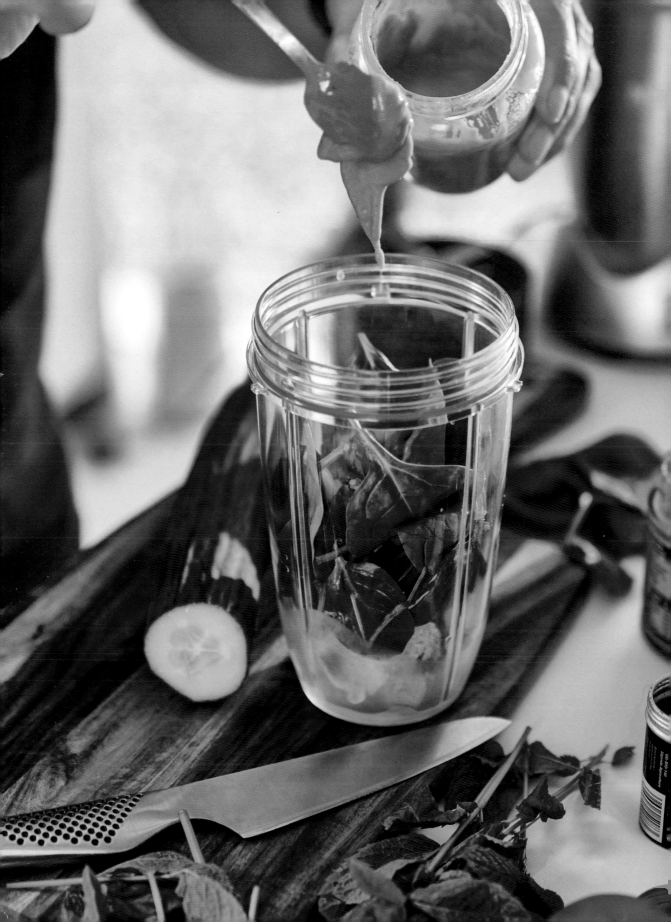

The Global
NUTRIBULLET
PHENOMENON

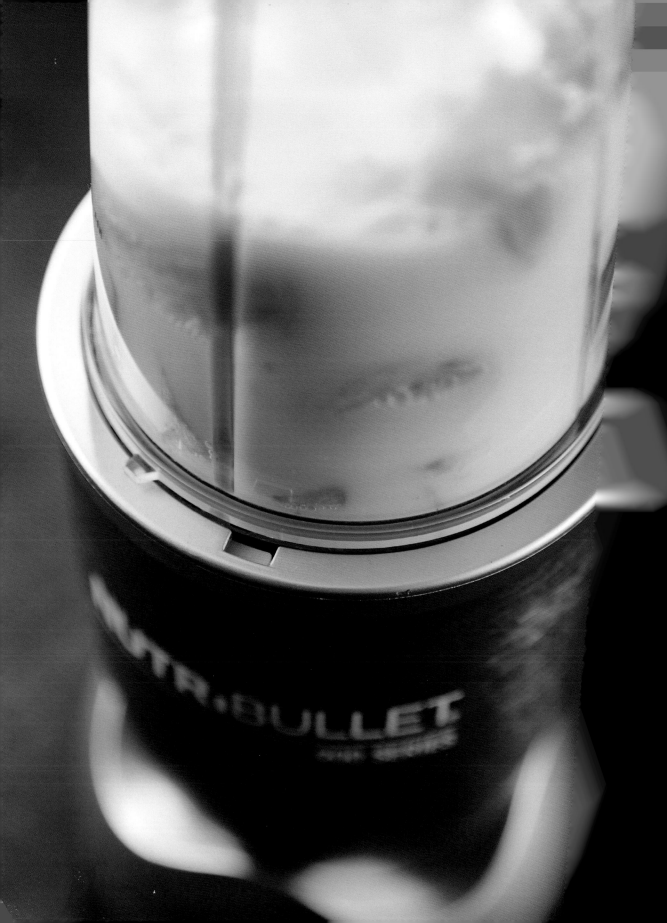

THE GLOBAL NUTRIBULLET PHENOMENON

Ever heard of the NutriBullet? Silly question really, as chances are,
not only have you heard of it, but with one being sold every
25 seconds, you probably have one in your kitchen right now!

T he NutriBullet phenomenon is exactly that, a *phenomenon*. Every now
and then, a product comes along which defines the expression, 'total
game-changer' (like the George Foreman grill a few years back) and
the NutriBullet has been, and continues to be, one of those products. They
have even gone on to raise the blending game further, with the world's first
smart bullet, or NutriBullet Balance, as it's officially known. This little beauty
not only makes the finest blends, but also hooks up to your smartphone or
tablet and tells you how much protein, fat and carbs are in your blend, as well
as how many calories – genius!

I genuinely believe the NutriBullet has been more responsible for the increase in
people's fruit and vegetable consumption than any other product on earth. Well, I
say more fruits *and* vegetables, but I really mean just fruit. The majority of people
with one of these blenders are usually using it primarily for fruit smoothies, the
vegetables have usually gone begging! This is mainly due to many people not
having the faintest idea of what (and how much) they should be blending, in order
to get lean and healthy. Because of this, there are many people out there blending
away who can't understand why they are still overweight and unhealthy, despite
consuming what they feel are healthy blends. It's because many are using their
blender in the wrong way and blitzing up blends which can rival the calorie content
of a McDonald's burger, fries *and* milkshake! Admittedly, it also didn't help that
the first recipe book that came with the NutriBullet featured recipes which just
didn't work and many were enough to put you off ever adding vegetables to your
blends again. I am absolutely convinced that whoever wrote the recipes in the
original book never actually made them, because some were totally undrinkable!
You cannot put three large carrots, two sticks of celery, half a cucumber, a handful
of spinach, two apples, a pear and some water into a NutriBullet and get a *nice*
drink, or 'NutriBlast,' as they call them. In fact, you won't get a drink from that
concoction at all. What you will end up with is a large mound of mush which will
be easier eaten with a spoon than drunk through a straw!

One of the reasons people were immediately attracted to the NutriBullet was because, unlike a juicer, it is much, *much* easier to clean. However, there are some things which belong in your juicer and should never venture into your bullet or blender, and vice versa.

Those who know my work will know I am a huge juicing advocate. I am, after all, known as the *Juice* Master. However, those who have read my juicing books and followed my plans will be fully aware that I have always included blending as part of my programmes, too. In my health documentary, *Super Juice Me!* (free to watch on YouTube, Amazon Prime and superjuiceme. com), blending played a 50% role in proceedings – with an avocado blend pretty much making a showing every morning and evening. This is why I am as equally passionate about blending, as I am juicing. I am also extremely passionate about making sure people use both machines in the right way and only juice what should be juiced and blend what should be blended.

When I set out over two decades ago to *Juice The World*, my main aim was to make a juicer and blender as common as a kettle and toaster in every household across the world. Two decades on, and more people

have juicers than ever in history, but far more have blenders – or a NutriBullet, to be more specific. It has also been shown that people are more likely to use a blender than a juicer, and this is largely down to the cleaning aspect. This is why, I believe, over the past few years in particular, I have literally been inundated with requests from people to devise a plant-protein-based blend plan, for sheer speed and ease.

So, I have taken my two plus decades' worth of experience in this area, and come up with a *pure blend* plan for those who wouldn't do a plan at all if they had to clean a juicer. I also wanted to devise a plan for people who aren't exactly enamoured by the earthy vegetable juice side of life and are looking for a good, plant-based protein plan.

MY MISSION IN THIS BOOK IS TWOFOLD:

1. Get you blending in the right way.

2. Provide you with the full *Super Blend Me!* programme – designed to get you: Super Lean – Super Healthy – Super Fast.

So, on with my first mission of getting you to use your blender the right way.

I have a clear and invaluable piece of advice to help you towards this goal:

DO NOT DRINK ANY BLEND FASTER THAN IT WOULD HAVE TAKEN YOU TO EAT THE RAW INGREDIENTS IN THAT BLEND

I will elaborate much more on this point as part of the *7 Rules For Success (page 59)*, later in the book (in *Rule 3* to be more specific). However, I wanted to mention it off the bat here, as this is where most people go wrong when it comes to blending, and where the writers of the first NutriBullet recipe book also messed up! Just because a product can blend a stupid amount of hard fruits and vegetables at once, and just because we can drink the pulverised pulp it produces in a few minutes flat, it doesn't mean we should.

Not drinking any blend faster than it would have taken to eat the raw ingredients is a key rule to stick to, to ensure you don't burden your system with too much insoluble fibre – or just too much food in general. It doesn't matter how good the ingredients are going in; if you're over burdening your system with too much, your body's not going to react well.

My second mission, and arguably the most important, is to do whatever I can to encourage you to give a *Super Blend Me! Challenge* a go. There is no question that, even if you don't do the plan itself and just use this book to get the right blends into your body each day, you will undoubtedly feel healthier. However, it is nothing compared to how you will look and feel when you go 'blend exclusive' for a set period of time. I know it's always best to under-promise and over-deliver, but I cannot even begin to describe to you just how much better you will look and feel at the end of your personal *Super Blend Me! Challenge*. I say, your *personal* challenge, because although the maximum *Super Blend Me! Challenge* is 21 days, the plan has been designed so you can do 7, 10, 14 or, of course, the big 21 days – it's your call. The minimum, in order to really see and feel noticeable results is 7 days, which is why I don't suggest anything less. A little FYI, if you decide to do the 10-day *Super Blend Me! Challenge*, you'll see monumental changes in a very short space of time.

When you eliminate *all* heavily processed food / drinks, and have only plant-based nutrition going into your body for a period of time, something truly remarkable happens. I realise this is now starting to sound a little 'praise the blend, it's a miracle', but I am so excited by this plan and cannot urge you enough to try this bad boy on for size.

The biggest convincer, as always, is seeing the results of *real* people: those who have tried and tested the plan and experienced the incredible results for themselves. If we're honest, all you really want to know when deciding on whether you will embark on a challenge like this is, does it work? And the answer, without any shadow of doubt, is a resounding YES – on *every* single level. You'll drop weight (if you need to), have more energy, feel healthier and have a razor-sharp, clear mind. I know this because I have personally done the 21-day *Super Blend Me! Challenge* (yes, I went for the big one; well I had to fully test it, after all!) and all of those things happened and more (and bear in mind I felt pretty good before I even started!).

However, you don't need to take my word for it, because I took a bunch of people of all shapes, sizes and sexes and put my *Super Blend Me!* plan to the test. I put some on the 7-day, some on the 10-day, some on the 14-day and some on the full 21-day challenge. I knew the results would be pretty good, after all, I have been doing this for over two decades and it's the only subject I know anything about. However, when I saw one guy had dropped 19lbs during the 10-day trial, I knew I was onto something really special with this plan. I will share some of the truly inspiring results from the trial in a sec – as chances are, they alone will be all that's needed to convince you to try a *Super Blend Me! Challenge* on for size – but one thing I need you to know, is that it doesn't matter who you are or what health / weight/ shredding goals you have, *Super Blend Me!* is...

A Plan
DESIGNED
for
EVERYONE

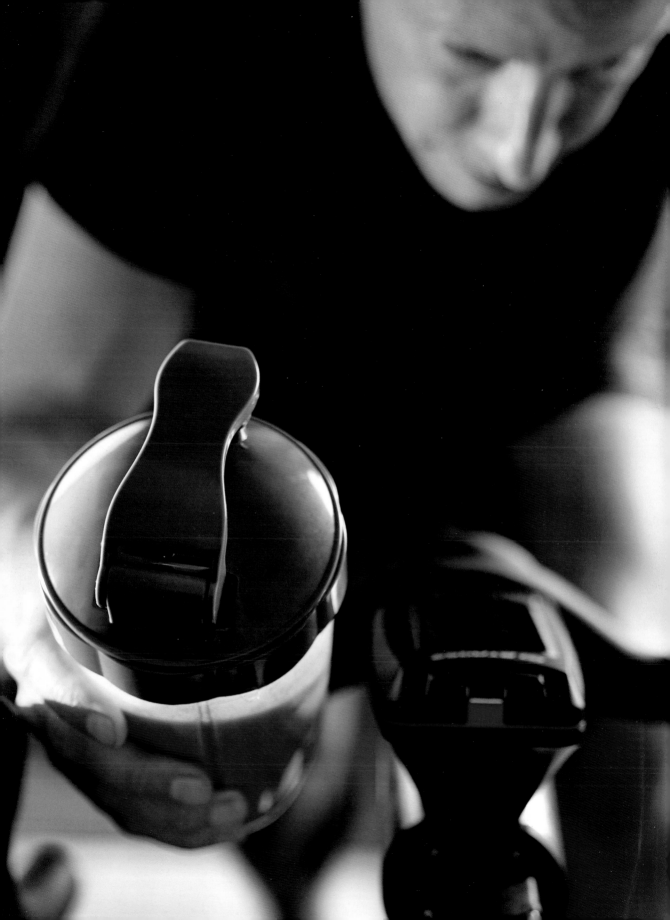

Super Blend Me! has been cleverly designed with everyone in mind. It doesn't matter if you have an enormous amount of weight to lose or you just want to get shredded — Super Blend Me! has the perfect amount of macronutrients (protein, fat and carbohydrates) as well as a plethora of micronutrients (vitamins, minerals and phytonutrients) to satiate and sustain you, whatever your lifestyle.

All the recipes have been balanced perfectly on the calorie front too. As you know, generally I am not a calorie person, but it's very easy to overdo it when making blends, so I've also taken a little nod in the calorie direction on this occasion (so you don't have to).

Super Blend Me!, due to its rich plant-protein-based recipes, has also been designed with exercise in mind. Whether you're an athlete or just someone who likes to exercise daily, you can exercise till your heart's content on this programme. To give you some idea, when I did the 21-day *Super Blend Me! Challenge,* I also decided to commit to cycling 21 miles on a spinning bike, for 21 days straight. I consistently beat my time every week, so if you're concerned that by taking part in the plan you won't have any energy to exercise, my results speak for themselves:

Week 1 21 miles in 58 minutes 12 seconds
Week 2 21 miles in 57 minutes 32 seconds
Week 3 21 miles in 53 minutes 55 seconds

Also, do not fear you'll lose muscle mass either, as the *Super Blend Me! Challenge* has been designed with amino acids in mind, the building blocks for protein. When you read some of the results from the test group, you'll see just how many people lost body fat but gained muscle mass. It could be easily argued that all protein ultimately comes from plants, as the largest land animals in the world are all vegan, and everything from a rhino to a fully-grown bull elephant gets *all* of their protein from the amino acids...found in *plants.* You've only got to look at the sheer muscle mass of a giraffe, bullock, elephant or even cow for that matter, to relax in the knowledge you'll be good to go on the protein front when getting your amino acids from plant-based foods. If you are a meat / dairy eater, you can relax in the knowledge that my intention for this book is not to turn you into a vegetarian or vegan come the end of this book. I simply want to point out that you don't need to worry about your protein intake for the duration of your *Super Blend Me! Challenge* – nature has it covered!

SUPER-CONVENIENT, SUPER-SATISFYING, SUPER-SPEEDY, SUPER-EASY

Super Blend Me! has also been designed with satisfaction, speed and convenience at its forefront. I wanted each recipe to not only taste really good and fully satisfy on the hunger front, but I also wanted them to be super-fast to make. I also didn't want to go too 'Instagram' with the ingredients. What I mean by that is, all of the recipes have been designed with genuine, sustained nutrition in mind, rather than using 'designer' ingredients to look all 'Instagramy' and 'Notting Hilly!' I'm all for using different ingredients, just not for the sake of it, or because someone's decided they're 'on trend'. The clean-eating Insta crowd always seem to be discovering a new berry, root or seed of some kind, and when they do, the impression is given that you'll perish or age prematurely unless you start consuming them in copious amounts. Chia seeds, turmeric, maca and charcoal are the 'on trend' ingredients at the time of writing of this, but you won't find any of them in this plan. I agree they are all good for you, but they won't add anything more to the recipes than is already there. Each recipe, as mentioned, has macro and micronutrients, as well as being loaded with antioxidants and phytonutrients. Each recipe also has natural anti-inflammatory ingredients, so nothing is to be gained by adding the trendy nutrition kids on the block into the plan just for the sake of being *on trend*. The only nutritional supplement essential to the plan (in addition to what I deem to be normal, everyday ingredients) is some plant-based protein powder, but even that is available pretty much everywhere now. Having said that, I do also suggest adding some *Super Blend Me! Greens* or *Super Blend Me! Berry* powders into some of the recipes, but please note these are completely optional. The reason for suggesting these additional powders is simply to add more micronutrients (vitamins, minerals and phytonutrients) to the plan. *Super Blend Me!* is already rich in macronutrients (proteins, fats and carbohydrates) and whilst it also has sufficient micronutrients, these powders just help to raise the micronutrient game. I also don't know the quality of produce you will be using, so if the fruit and veg you buy isn't up to scratch, these powders will make up the nutritional shortfall. Once again, these are *optional* and you can rest in the knowledge that the main and most important ingredients are simple everyday items, that are widely available to all.

WASTE NOT, WANT NOT

I not only wanted to use as many simple everyday ingredients as possible, but also to make the plan even more convenient and economical, by repeating some of the key ingredients (in different combinations) throughout the plan. I also wanted to make sure you're not buying ingredients you are only going to use once (the only exception to this are the three *Special Guest* recipes) and I didn't want anything to really mess with the flavours. I find maca powder, for example, can ruin the flavour of a good blend, and turmeric can also do the same. This doesn't mean I don't ever have blends with these wonderful ingredients in, or that there aren't ways to make them taste good, because there are, I just wanted to keep this as simple and as recognisable for everyone as possible. For instance, you may know what maca is if you're a

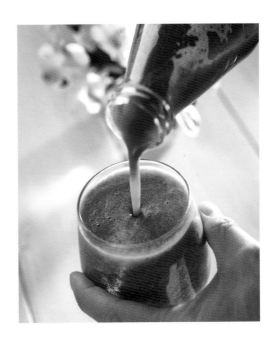

30-year-old living in London, but if you're 70-year-old who lives in a small country village, you may not have a Scooby Doo (that's Cockney rhyming slang for clue!). I've also made absolutely sure that each *Super Blend* is balanced nutritionally, tastes amazing and adheres to my key blending principle of not containing too much insoluble fibre.

THE 'JUICE PLAN' FOR PEOPLE WHO 'DON'T DO JUICE PLANS'

Super Blend Me! has been described as the 'juice plan for people who don't do juice plans' (stay with me!) There are a few things that can put certain people off ever doing a juice 'detox' and cleaning the juicer is, without question, at number one. Personally, I don't mind, I'm used to it, and it actually takes less time than people think. I also know the huge benefits of juicing outweigh the slight inconvenience of cleaning the machine. However, there are some who see the cleaning process as a nightmare and simply refuse to get involved in a juice challenge because of it. Then there's the taste factor; as mentioned, these blends taste amazing, especially when comparing to some of the earthier juices. Many *pure* juice plans take quite a nod in the earthy direction taste-wise, which often can't be helped due to most being largely vegetable-based, but this can put some people off. Having said that, I have always made sure that the juice plans I devise also taste great too. There is a way to get the perfect balance of flavours when combining vegetable and fruit juices, but many get it wrong. I personally love the earthier juices, but I am aware there are many out there who wouldn't drink raw beetroot juice for all the tea in China, so this plan is perfect for them. The main beauty of *Super Blend Me!* though, is there's no juicer to clean, and a blender takes seconds to rinse through. There are also many ingredients which blend beautifully but don't work in your juicer. Nut butters, for example, not only create a wonderful creamy texture and taste but also add good amounts of protein, which helps to keep you satisfied. Blends are super-fast to make; in fact it shouldn't take you any longer than five minutes make each recipe, and this time *includes* the washing up!

Another huge blending perk is being able to take advantage of the convenience that comes from frozen produce, as there are many things which can be blended from frozen, but clearly not juiced, such as avocados, berries, spinach, kale, banana and even ginger. Being able to make the majority of your blends with ingredients from just your cupboard and freezer makes for one extremely convenient, no waste, quick and easy plan (see *Tip 2, Let Your Freezer and Cupboard Become Your Best Friends,* page 77).

THE DEFINITION OF 'DETOX'

I have also tried to eliminate, or at least tone down, any detox symptoms you may experience. The term 'detox' isn't strictly correct. There are many doctors, dieticians and nutritionists out there who still freak out when people use the term, especially when people say things like they are 'going on a detox'. The reason for this is that they argue we have perfectly good organs that do all the

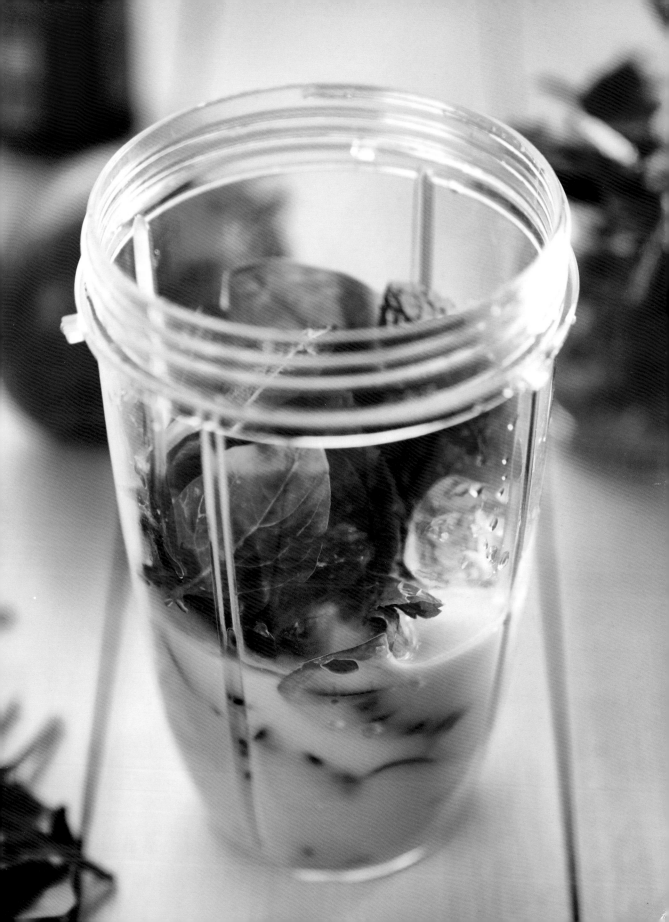

detoxing for us, such as the liver, skin, lungs, kidneys, etc., and that healthy foods / juices / blends, etc. are not capable of detoxing. This is true, and I wholeheartedly agree that only the body can 'detox' the body; however, what they fail to realise is that the new collective definition of the word 'detox' has changed. If you ask the average person in the street what 'going on a detox' means to them, the answer you will get 99.99% of the time is:

'ABSTAINING FROM UNHEALTHY FOODS OR DRINKS FOR A SET PERIOD OF TIME'

They haven't grasped that the *vast majority* of people understand 'detox' to simply mean a period of abstinence from junk foods and drinks, aka a period of time of consuming only healthy foods and drinks. Oh, and if you really want to rattle their pedantic cages, tell them you're doing a 'cleanse' – watch them really lose their crap! Oddly, one of the guys who gets extremely worked up about people using what he describes as 'misleading terms' like 'detox' and 'cleanse' was one of the founders of a company called The Food Doctor ... yes, *doctor* ... not misleading at all then! (It's a food *company* ... not a food *doctor*).

So, if you do ever happen to say to someone that you are 'on a detox' whilst doing your *Super Blend Me! Challenge* and they respond by telling you that it's only your organs that can in fact 'detox' you, please tell them to go get a life! It's amazing how some people get so caught up with such stupid semantics in order to try and gain some kind of significance, when everyone knows exactly what you really mean.

Having said that, although I do use expressions like 'on a detox' and 'detox symptoms', I tend to use a more accurate word when describing the symptoms you may experience during the first 72 hours of one of my plans, and that's – withdrawal. Yes, in reality, you won't be experiencing 'detox' symptoms at all, but rather *withdrawal* symptoms.

When you stop smoking you experience nicotine withdrawal, not nicotine detox. The same can happen when you suddenly stop things like refined fat, salt, sugar, caffeine and alcohol. It doesn't happen in every case, but some type of withdrawal is usually felt. However, because in the *Super Blend Me! Challenge* I have used plenty of delicious things like almond butter, cashew butter, bananas and avocados, any withdrawal you may feel should be significantly less than on a *juice only* plan. This is because good quality fat and protein (amino acids) help to regulate the appetite, whilst ingredients like bananas and dates will alleviate any sugar withdrawal you may have. Yes, some people *may* still get a headache and some *may* feel more tired than normal during the first couple of days, but the majority of people who trialled the plan reported that hunger wasn't an issue and their energy levels remained the same. So, if you do experience any withdrawal and you aren't feeling yourself, please know this will only be for the first 72 hours maximum, after which time the withdrawal will be over and you'll come out the other side feeling fresh and ready for anything.

If you do find your energy levels take a slight slump during the first 72 hours due to the withdrawal, then please listen to your body. The withdrawal from refined sugar, refined fats and things like artificial sweeteners and alcohol affect different people in different ways. Most people are okay and experience only slight withdrawal on the *Super Blend Me! Challenge*. However, if the norm for you is to rev yourself up with loads

of caffeine (whether through coffee or energy drinks) and loads of sugar (whether through cereals, bread, chocolate, muffins, crisps, etc.) you may come down to earth with a bit of a bump and adrenal fatigue may kick in. When a person frequently runs on what I describe as *false stimulants*, they tend to feel extremely tired the moment they eliminate these stimulants from their diet. I say *false stimulants*, because ultimately what goes up must come down. If you rev *up* your system with white refined sugar, caffeine, nicotine or artificial sweeteners, inevitably you will experience a come *down* of some nature. This is often adrenal fatigue caused, ironically, by these so-called stimulating foods and drinks. This is why I refer to them as *false stimulants* as in the end, for a person who constantly relies on these foods and drinks as their main pick-me-ups, all they are doing is trying to lift themselves from the adrenal fatigue low, caused by the last dose.

If you are a person who does use the aforementioned foods and drinks a great deal of the time (and, worryingly, there are some people who only consume these foods and drinks) then as mentioned, it usually takes a couple of days for the body to start tapping into its natural energy stores, so hang on in there. In fact, to put to bed any fears you may have, check out *The Incredible Results* chapter (page 35) as you will see the few trial candidates who experienced this 72-hour withdrawal period, came out the other side and were flying high by day four. Short-term discomfort for long-term pleasure!

If tiredness and fatigue does set in, then clearly listen to your body, rest as much as you can for the first couple of days and ease off the exercise. However, I will stress that most people are good to go on the exercise front from day one, but just use your head and listen to your body.

Like I said earlier, I chose to cycle 21 miles on a spinning bike from day one, but on day two, I did feel a slight slump in energy and had to have a very early night! After a good night's sleep, my energy soon picked up and I noticed a significant increase in my energy levels from day four onwards. When you read the results later, you'll read a couple of times that, 'the first three days were tricky, but by day four I was flying'. I personally believe that they would have had a much easier ride if they'd just listened to their bodies and understood that…

The Main
WITHDRAWAL
is in the
MIND

THE FREEDOM THINKING TECHNIQUE

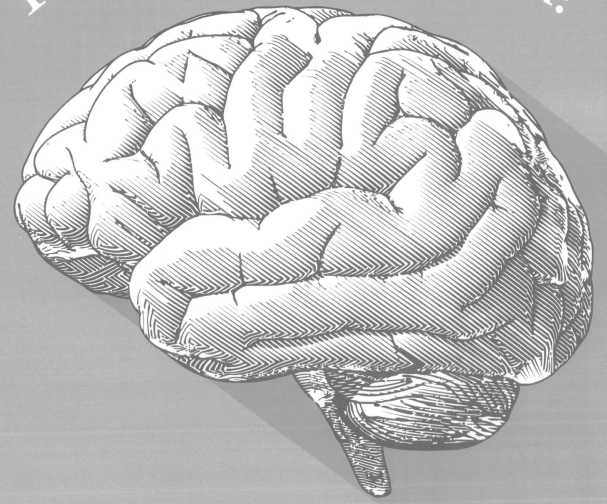
It's All In The Mind!

The main withdrawal is not actually felt in the body, but rather very much in the mind. If anything is going to break you and stop you from completing your Super Blend Me! Challenge, it's the psychological withdrawal from certain foods and drinks; not the physical symptoms.

P hysically, in real nutrition terms, you aren't actually being deprived of anything. I have, as mentioned, made sure that the *Super Blend Me!* plan meets all of your nutritional needs. So, it's not the physical withdrawal, but rather a feeling of *mental deprivation* that can cause a person to break. Luckily, this is easily dealt with. It is just a case of an extremely simple, yet unbelievably powerful, shift in thinking. It is the switch from *diet* thinking to *freedom* thinking and it really can be the difference between success and failure.

If you have ever read any of my *juice* plan books, you will know that I have always focused a great deal on mindset. We can't underestimate the often extremely psychological addictive pull of certain foods and drinks, and how difficult some people can find it to let go of these, even if it's just for 7–21 days. The main foods and drinks people struggle to say farewell to, for any length of time, are those loaded with white refined sugar, refined fats and, of course, for many – alcohol.

The good news is, as mentioned previously, any genuine physical withdrawal from these foods or drinks usually only lasts for around 72 hours. Most of these you won't even notice on the *Super Blend Me! Challenge* anyway due, as mentioned, to the good fat, protein and natural sugar content of the specially devised *Super Blends*. However, the psychological withdrawal, that feeling of *mental* deprivation, of missing out on what others are having, can last the entire duration of your challenge if you don't make a significant shift in your thinking.

So, if you find yourself getting a little snappy with others, or even very irate during the first few days, this will most likely not be caused by any real physical discomfort from the 'detox'. You might feel a little tired or get a headache as mentioned, but you need to realise that your snappy mood is most likely being caused by what is going on inside your own head. The truth is, the mind is extremely powerful, and whether you find the *Super Blend Me! Challenge* easy or difficult will be largely down to how you approach it mentally every day.

MAKE IT EASY ON YOURSELF!

There's always an easy way and a hard way to approach most things; oddly, when it comes to a 'detox' or dieting, most opt for the hard way. The only reason they choose the hard option is twofold:

1. **The vast majority of people approach it in exactly the same way and so think this must be the way to do it.**

2. **They just don't know the simple mind shift which can change the game entirely.**

This is why I have included the incredibly simple *Freedom Thinking Technique* in this book and, why I am so adamant you read the whole book before starting (excluding the *Congratulations You've Done It* and *Life After Super Blend Me!* sections, which should be read on your final day). It is much easier to get in the right shape of body, if you first get into the right frame of mind. You may feel you don't need any coaching and you've got this covered, but please, humour me! I have been doing this for over two decades, and I know that a simple shift in your mental approach can make all the difference. And when I talk about helping you to get into the right frame of mind, I am not talking about willpower – this is the common approach and is deeply flawed. Mainly because, more often than not, the stronger willed you tend to be, the harder you will find it, if you're using willpower as the only method to 'get you through'. No, that's not a typo, and yes, you did read correctly:

The stronger willed you are, the more difficult you will find your *Super Blend Me! Challenge* if you are using willpower as your main psychological tool to complete it.

Imagine this. There's two children who are about to tuck into their favourite chocolate bar. One is strong-willed and one is weak-willed. They both really want the chocolate bar, and are about to take their first bite when their mother comes in, tells them they have to wait until after tea, and takes the chocolate bars away. Who do you think will kick up more of a fuss? Bizarrely, the strong-willed child, as the weak-willed child will accept the situation a lot sooner. Willpower is *only needed* if you are trying to stop yourself from having something you really want or desire. If both the strong-willed child and weak-willed child had zero desire for the chocolate and you took the bars away, who would kick up more of a fuss then? Neither of them! Why? Because neither child has any desire or want for the chocolate, so it's completely irrelevant whether they are strong or weak-willed. Willpower, to repeat the point, only comes into play when you are trying to stop yourself having something you want or desire. If you remove the want or desire, you remove the need for willpower – it's that simple.

THERE'S NO NEED TO 'WHITE-KNUCKLE-RIDE' IT

Therefore, the key to making your *Super Blend Me! Challenge* not only easy, but also enjoyable, so you actually complete it, is to manage your thoughts effectively. As previously highlighted, this is where most get it wrong and it's where many, if they are going to cave in, cave. Most people's attempts to complete a plan of this nature, are flawed from the get go. They not only *start* with feelings of dread and deprivation, but they tend to 'white-knuckle-ride' the whole way through…or until the point of failure. What I mean is, they not only start by forcing themselves into a self-imposed mental tantrum a great deal of the time, but they also spend the entire time just 'hanging on in there', taking one day at a time and hoping things will get easier. The madness, of course, is they are the ones making it

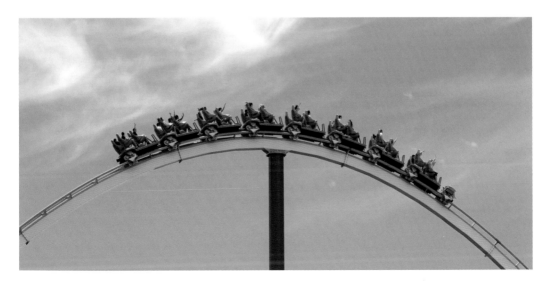

difficult for themselves, no one else! And the main thing that they are doing, which is making it a million times harder than it ever needs to be, is the biggest madness of all:

THEY ARE CONSTANTLY MOPING AROUND FOR FOODS AND DRINKS WHICH THEY HOPE THEY WON'T HAVE!

They are in a tantrum because they feel they *can't* have certain foods or drinks, but this is madness for two reasons:

1. The *Super Blend Me! Challenge* is only from 7, up to a maximum of 21 days. So, whatever they feel they're missing out on; it's very temporary.

2. They can have whatever they want, whenever they want!

Think about it. Nothing is actually preventing them from grabbing a sandwich / chocolate / some crisps / a beer / glass of wine or whatever they want, whenever they choose; they are adults, after all. What they forget is, they are *choosing* to do the plan as they *want* the incredible results it will bring. They also seem to forget that the foods and drinks they think they are missing out on, are the very things which caused whatever weight gain or health problems they so desperately hate living with. So, the last thing they actually want is to throw in the towel early, and they'd have a much better chance of not throwing in that towel if they just stopped driving themselves crazy with a 'can't' mentality and reminded themselves that they have a choice, they can have whatever they like, but are simply choosing not to.

THE FREEDOM OF GENUINE CHOICE

You need to remember that if you decide to take on a *Super Blend Me! Challenge*, it will be *your* choice, no one is forcing you to do it, so don't drive yourself cuckoo or make it a thousand times harder for yourself by constantly moping around for foods and drinks which, ironically, you hope you won't have! I caught myself doing this a couple of times when testing the plan. I started to feel deprived and kept focusing on what I *thought* I couldn't have. It then dawned on me that I could have whatever the hell I wanted, I'm an adult, after all, and no one was actually

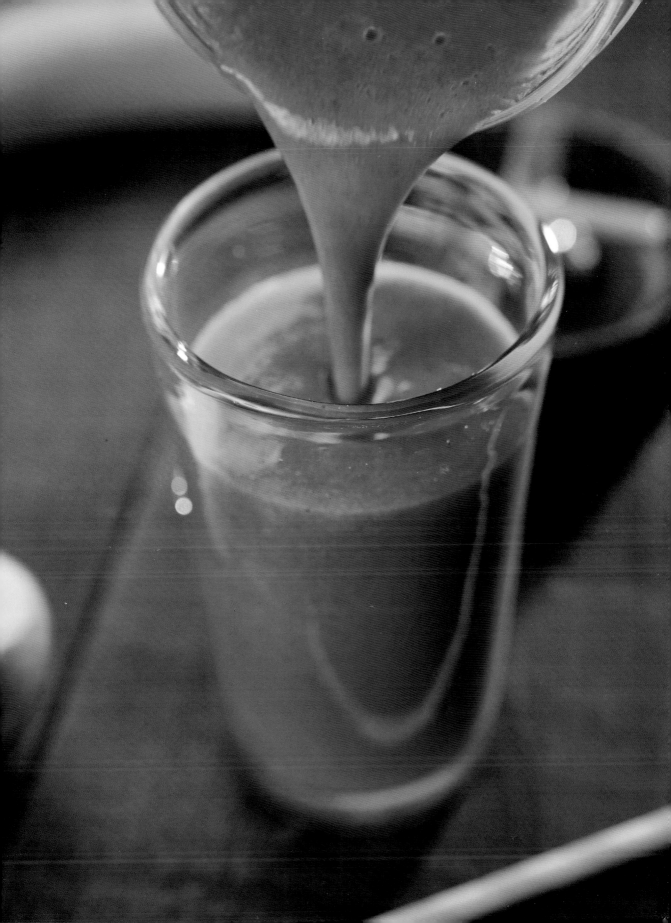

stopping me. It then dawned on me that if someone had actually handed me what I *thought* I wanted and what I was internally bitching about not having, I would have said no. At the end of the day, I had set myself a challenge and wanted to complete that challenge. I wanted to know how *Super Blend Me!* would make me feel and wanted the results I knew it would bring. I then took some of my own *correct thinking* medicine and opted for some straight talking:

'EITHER HAVE IT AND SHUT UP OR DON'T HAVE IT AND SHUT UP, BUT WHATEVER YOU DO, SHUT UP!'

You simply need to shift your mind from a diet mentality of **'I WANT, BUT I CAN'T HAVE'** to **'I CAN HAVE, BUT I DON'T WANT'**.

This easy shift in the thinking, if adopted correctly, is far more powerful than its simplicity suggests. I was bitching because I felt I couldn't have something that, in real terms, I clearly could. The second I said to myself, 'Either have it and shut up or don't have it and shut up, but whatever you do, Jason – SHUT UP!' I was okay. Years ago, I thought of an acronym for the word *can't*, in relation to a dieting situation and, although I've mentioned it in other books, just in case this is your first *Jason book* outing, here it is again:

CONSTANT **A**ND **N**EVER-ending **T**ANTRUM

People often force themselves into a self-imposed mental tantrum, akin to a child kicking up a fuss, if they feel deprived. However, once again, and to really hammer this point home for the final time, to ensure you really take it on board to make your *Super Blend Me! Challenge* a breeze:

THE MAJORITY OF 'SUFFERING' WHEN EMBARKING ON ANY DIET / DETOX / CHALLENGE OF THIS NATURE IS NOT CAUSED BY ANY GENUINE PHYSICAL DEPRIVATION BUT RATHER A FEELING OF MENTAL DEPRIVATION.

IN OTHER WORDS, WHETHER YOU FIND IT EASY OR DIFFICULT LIES FIRMLY AT YOUR OWN THINKING DOOR!

Some are quick to forget that they *want* the incredible results the challenge will bring. Others feel like they are having to make many sacrifices when doing a 'detox', forgetting the *huge* sacrifices they make on a daily basis, by not doing it. I used to be overweight and sick on many levels, and the sacrifices I had to make on a daily basis far exceeded any 'sacrifices' I made on my journey to getting fit and healthy.

THE SACRIFICES YOU CONSTANTLY MAKE BY NOT CHANGING ARE THE ONES YOU NEED TO WORRY ABOUT!

The irony, of course, is that most people who will be embarking on a *Super Blend Me! Challenge* will already be genuinely deprived of so many things and, as a result, are already making huge sacrifices every day of their lives. If you don't have the energy you want, the body you want, the health you want, the level of fitness you want – you are being deprived. We never really look at how much *not* making a change costs us in every area of our lives. At the time of writing this book I am approaching 50 years old, and this morning I jumped on a spinning bike for a 45-minute blast, bounced for 20 minutes on a mini-trampoline and then jumped in the river for a swim. I then spent the morning sorting out a bit of business at my health retreat in Portugal and now I'm spending the afternoon writing this book. I also haven't taken a single medical drug for any lifestyle disease, or used a medical-based cream or potion for over twenty years, and honestly, I feel better today than I did when I was 18. Why? Because back then I was obese, covered in a skin disease, had severe asthma, hay fever, was taking medical drugs, smoking like a chimney, drinking like a fish, eating nothing but junk and was constantly tired (shocker!). It was during the time when I ate / drank the rubbish and didn't exercise that I sacrificed the most. I had to make sacrifices in every single area of my life, from not being able to wear what I wanted, to not having the energy to play the game I adore most in the world – football. I also had to make sacrifices in relationships (not many women were keen on a fat, skin-diseased heavy smoker and drinker – funny, that) as well as in my social and work life. I was literally existing, having half a life and being deprived of the pure, genuine energy you get from a good nutritious diet and moving your body.

So, if you originally thought that you'd have to make sacrifices in order to embark on a *Super Blend Me! Challenge*, take a moment to really think about every area of your life where you're already making genuine sacrifices, without even realising it. From the clothes you can't fit into, the illnesses you may suffer from that hold you back, to the energy you don't have to allow you to really embrace the opportunities life has to offer. Also, take a moment to focus on the fact that this is only for a very short space of time (even if you pick the maximum 21-day challenge) and really consider what can be achieved in the short-term, that you can benefit from long-term. Rest in the knowledge that the best part of *Super Blend Me!* is how it resets your mind and body. Give *Super Blend Me!* a minimum of seven days to work its full magic, and come day eight, the last thing you'll want is junk; you'll actually be craving healthy stuff. This is why so many people who did the trial carried on *after* they had finished. It was the catalyst they had been looking for to essentially reprogramme their mind and body and turn that mental switch from wanting junk to genuinely wanting the good stuff.

THE PROOF OF THE PUDDING IS IN THE . . . BLENDING!

I am, of course, aware that many who choose to do a *Super Blend Me! Challenge* will already have their healthy s**t together. This is my first plant-protein-based plan, and so I know it will appeal to many gym bunnies and those who already exercise regularly and eat pretty well. At the same time, I know that there will be many people who are desperate to get their healthy s**t together and who are desperate to drop some weight, sort out some of their health issues and reset their exercise mojo. As I have said, *Super Blend Me!* has been designed for *everyone*, no matter what end of the scale you are. This is why for the trial I chose a cross section of people, from fairly lean athletes to those who had huge weight and health challenges.

As the main aim of this book is to inspire you to try a *Super Blend Me! Challenge* on for size, which, in turn, will help to reset your mind and body for a healthier way of life, I see no reason in delaying sharing a nice selection of results from said trial. I could spend many pages waxing lyrical about the nutritional benefits of the *Super Blends*, or how best to use the *Freedom Thinking Technique* to make it easy, but when push comes to shove, let's face facts, nothing will convince you more than...

The
INCREDIBLE
RESULTS

I DROPPED 10LBS IN 7 DAYS!

LOST 19LBS (8.6KG)
IN 10 DAYS!

LOST 3% BODY FAT!

MUSCLE INCREASED 3%

LOST 11.5LBS (5.2KG) IN 7 DAYS!
LOST 4CM OFF HIPS

OVER 4% REDUCTION IN BODY FAT

When it came to testing Super Blend Me! – there was no shortage of volunteers. I put a small post on my Facebook page, and in just 24 hours we had over 3,000 people apply to be part of the trial. I think the reason for such interest was partly due to this being my first plant-protein-based plan, and partly due to the fact they knew they wouldn't have to clean a juicer!

What you need to know about the trials I conduct is that I always like them to be as real as possible. I don't buy the fruit and veg for those taking part, nor do I make the *Super Blends* for them, and I certainly don't hold their hand along the way. The trial conditions are the same as if the person had just got the book or the app and were following the plan at home, so are completely left to their own devices. It's worth noting that because the book hadn't been fully written when the test group did their challenges, you're actually in a much better position than they were. Not only do you have the benefit of an improved plan, due to the tweaks made as a result of feedback from the trial group (for example, you'll never have to taste the first version of the *Tahini Protein Berry Blast*, which you'll be very pleased about!) but, because of the trial, you also get to see the sorts of amazing results that can be achieved, before you start. In addition, you have the benefit of the simple but extremely effective *Freedom Thinking Technique*, which helps more than many often give it credit for. If you have the Super Blend Me! app, you'll also be able to take advantage of the plethora of videos, including *the 7 Tips* and *7 Rules For Success*, which I've added some meat to. None of this was available to the people taking part in the trial and yet, as you will see, they still achieved off the scale, stupid results and enjoyed their journey.

READ THE RESULTS AND BREATHE THEM IN

Please don't just skip or scan-read through the results, they are a very important part of your mental preparation for the challenge, so take the time to fully take them on board and absorb the sheer magnitude of what you are reading. It is highly likely, after all, that the results you are about to read will be your biggest motivation to not only try a *Super Blend Me! Challenge*.

PAUL B

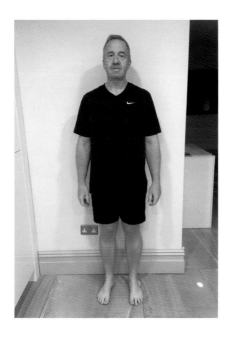

"I feel fantastic: lighter, cleaner, more energetic. Friends and family have commented how sparkly my eyes look and how trim I am!"

LOST 16lbs (7.3kg) IN 14 DAYS
BODY FAT REDUCED 3%
MUSCLE INCREASED 1%

Hi Jason and Co,
I've completed the 14 days but am travelling with work at the moment and have left my feedback forms at home – doh! Once I've got my dear wife to send them through, I'll get them to you over the next couple of days. Headlines, though, are: lost 16lbs in 14 days, body fat down by nearly 3% and muscle mass up by nearly 1%. Feel great and will continue with a combination of juices, blends, low HI meals and the odd bowl of ice cream...!"
Paul B

MY THOUGHTS . . .

First up, let's not ignore the big headline here, a 16lb weight loss in just 14 days. Yes, you heard right, that's **SIXTEEN POUNDS** or **7.3 KILOS** (the equivalent of eight bags of sugar!). That's a huge amount of weight to drop in such a short space of time. I wish to emphasise that Paul had the weight to lose, which is partly why the weight loss was so large, but there's no way he would have got anywhere near this sort of weight loss on a normal 'calorie-controlled diet'. However, for me the 16lb weight loss isn't the main story here (although I'm sure Paul would disagree!). It's the fact he **reduced** his body fat and **increased** his muscle mass. Many people wrongly assume that unless you are eating loads of animal protein, or having what's deemed as enough calories, you'll automatically lose muscle mass, gain more actual fat and have no energy. Paul did an average of an hour's exercise each day, whilst having just three *Super Blends* each day and yet he not only **lost** body fat and gained muscle, but his energy also increased. Well, I say the main story here is the reduced body fat and muscle gain, but Paul's journey to better health and body shape didn't start here. Coincidentally, as I write this, Paul has just turned up at my Juicy Oasis retreat in Portugal. We got talking on one of the morning walks, where he not only told me about his extremely positive *Super Blend Me! Challenge* experience, but how his journey had actually started back in January, when he first came to my juice retreat. He lost a whopping 14lbs in a week, continued on his health journey afterwards, and then did the *Super Blend Me!* trial where, as you know, he dropped a further 16lbs. All in all, since kicking off his health journey, Paul has lost a total of 56lbs (25 kilos) – that's a life-changing amount of weight loss. There are those who view juice / blend plans of this nature as quick fixes, but I have met many 'Pauls' over the past twenty years of doing this, who got so motivated by their initial results that it acted as a catalyst for lifelong change. I would say, no matter what weight you have to lose or health challenges you want to get to grips with, try a *Super Blend Me! Challenge* on for size – it just may change everything!

GARETH W

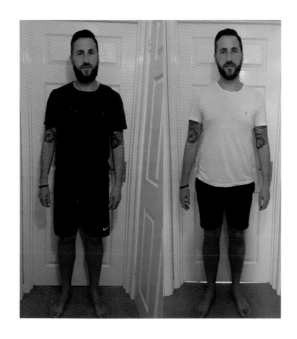

"I lost 19lbs,
2 inches off my
waist and hips,
3 inches off my
chest and had over
a 4% reduction
in my body fat."

LOST 19lbs (8.6kg) IN 10 DAYS
LOST 5cm OFF WAIST & HIPS
LOST 7.5cm OFF CHEST
4% REDUCTION IN BODY FAT

"What an amazing experience!! Thanks for choosing me... The best thing about the whole experience for me is how much clearer my mind feels and how much more energetic I feel. The plan was easy to follow and the preparation and clean-up is minimal. The smoothies all taste great... the energy I gained allowed me to cycle 16k a day and continue to play football which, at the start of the plan, I wasn't expecting to be able to do on blends alone. On the penultimate night of my 10-day challenge I went food shopping and the thought of eating chocolate or fatty foods just didn't appeal to me anymore. I intend to follow the 5:2 blend plan following this. Thank you so much again for choosing me."
Gareth W

MY THOUGHTS . . .

This was the first set of results to come in from the 10-day test group, and when I saw Gareth's, I think I re-read them about ten times to make sure I wasn't seeing things! This dude dropped **19lbs in 10 days** – that's **NINETEEN POUNDS**! That's almost **NINE KILOS** – that's a serious amount of weight. That's the sort of weight loss that really inspires people and the sort of weight loss that creates incredible positive momentum. We currently live in a completely insane world, when it comes to apparently healthy weight loss government guidelines. It seems you can gain as much weight as you like in a week, but believe it or not, current guidelines say it isn't healthy to lose more than 2lbs. I am not kidding either. If you gained 19lbs in 10 days by massively overeating on junk and not exercising, people wouldn't freak out anywhere near as much than if you dropped 19lbs in a week consuming plant-based nutrition and moving your body. I say 'people', but what I really mean are some state registered dieticians, as well as some doctors and 'nutritionists'. We are currently in the grasp of an obesity, diabetes and health crisis, and yet whenever anyone drops a significant amount of weight in a short space of time, all hell breaks loose! The arguments they usually level at this sort of rapid weight loss are twofold:

1. The 19lbs lost isn't all fat, it's mainly water.
2. The person will regain this weight just as rapidly as they lost it when they go back to normal eating.

Firstly, clearly Gareth didn't lose 19lbs of pure fat in the 10 days of *Super Blend Me!* – no one said he did. It is actually scientifically impossible to do so, unless you get it sucked out! However, he did drop 19lbs of something over the course of 10 days, as part of his body 'cleaning house', and as a result, he is 19lbs lighter. His body finally had the time, space and the right tools to 'clean house' effectively and it started the process with gusto. It's like if you had a bath full of utterly filthy water with fat floating around and you pulled the plug out, it would all disappear down the plughole in a very short space of time – not just the fat. The body wants to heal and will do so as quickly as it has the space, time and tools to do so. If Gareth started the plan at a normal weight and lost 19lbs in 10 days, then yes, there would be cause for great concern. As it is, he had this weight to lose (starting at almost 15 stone / 210lbs) and therefore this significant, rapid drop in weight is a very good thing. You will also notice his body fat reduced by 4%!

Secondly, the argument about gaining all the weight back when the person goes back to normal eating all depends on your definition of 'normal'. Gareth started his *Super Blend Me!* journey weighing in at a rather large 14 stone 13lbs. It was his 'normal' diet that led to him being that size, so obviously if he were to go back to his 'normal' way of eating, he'd soon gain all the weight back again – but what on earth has that got to do with his amazing weight loss success on the *Super Blend Me!* plan? If he were to go back to his old way of eating and gain all the weight back, it clearly wouldn't be because the plan didn't work, but rather because he started eating crap again. I say 'clearly', but sadly this point isn't clear to many, including some over 'qualified' dieticians and nutritional 'professionals'. Many will also often argue that when the person goes back to normal eating, not only will they gain the weight back, but they'll also gain more than before they started the 'diet'. What they don't seem to fathom is that if, for example, a person was gaining weight month on month, year on year, as a result of their normal diet before doing a plan like *Super Blend Me!* then isn't it painfully obvious, to all that if they return to their old normal, they'll gain the weight back (and then some!). They were gaining all the time before, so clearly they'll continue to gain weight if they return to that normal diet.

What many of the professionals in charge of the nation's health and guidelines don't fully grasp is that nothing inspires a person to carry on more, than significant results in the early stages. If Gareth had dropped 3lbs on the 10-day *Super Blend Me! Challenge* (which current guidelines insist is all that's healthy to lose) instead of the 19lbs he actually lost, I can guarantee he wouldn't have been anywhere near as psyched to continue. I also feel the most impressive and telling comment from his feedback was:

"On the penultimate night of my 10-day challenge I went food shopping and the thought of eating chocolate or fatty foods just didn't appeal to me anymore. I intend to follow the 5:2 Blend plan following this. Thank you so much again for choosing me."

This, above all else, is the real beauty of *Super Blend Me!* – when you finish, you don't want the crap anymore and you crave the good stuff. In fact, in virtually all trial cases, although they could clearly have anything they wanted the morning after the trial was over, most still chose to have a blend for breakfast. It is also interesting to observe how, by the end of the challenge, the thought of eating chocolate and fatty foods just simply didn't appeal to Gareth any more. And isn't that the Holy Grail – to just not want the crap anymore and be perfectly happy and satisfied without it? To actually crave healthy foods so they become part of your normal diet, without any fear of deprivation? Gareth's mindset and biochemistry has changed and so has his normal diet. If he goes back to his old normal, he'll gain all the weight back and more. However, if he carries on embracing his new normal, then clearly he won't. We should never underestimate the power of positive momentum and those who complete a *Super Blend Me! Challenge*, especially if they do a 10-day one or more, will have bags of it by the end. I'm talking about extremely powerful, often long-term, life-changing, positive momentum, that you simply don't get from a standard 'drop 2lbs in a week calorie-controlled diet'.

TOM T

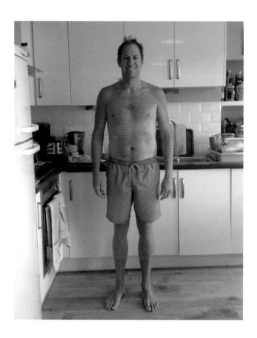

"The blends have been much more filling . . . I've exercised a lot but not felt hungry"

LOST 11.5lbs (5.2kg) IN 7 DAYS!
LOST 4cm OFF HIPS
LOST 3cm OFF WAIST
LOST 2cm OFF CHEST

"I have completed the Super Blend Me! 7-day Challenge & I will always use it as a preference to juicing. I love juicing, and will still do it as they taste amazing, but on any extended programme I often feel hungry, particularly when I exercise a lot. The blends have been much more filling, even though you have three instead of four. I assume the increased protein content is more filling. I have achieved similar weight loss on blends as with juices at Juicy Oasis. The fantastic thing about blends for me is the speed, it makes it much more practical in a busy family house to knock up a quick nutritious snack. This week I've exercised a lot but not felt hungry and not felt like I was overworking my body, this is great news. I preferred the thicker blends. Had my first blend at 10:30am., then the next two, four hours apart. It has been much easier to stick to than juicing whilst also being with the family and catering for

them all day. The hardest night was day seven as I was looking forward to eating again. Make sure you always have a proper blender, we only had a stick blender on a couple of days and the blends were a totally different texture. Very bitty. Your kids will love some of them, great way to get extra veg in them! Need to remember to combine more weights with my cardio work long term. I will continue with one or two blends a day!"
Tom T

MY THOUGHTS . . .

Tom lost a truly unbelievable 11.5lbs (5.2 kilos) in just seven days and a huge 3cm off his waist. Once again, these are quick, extremely noticeable results, which will make a person much more likely to carry on than if they'd only dropped a couple of pounds. As I expressed earlier, people want to see and feel as quickly as possible that what they are doing is getting results, and boy does a *Super Blend Me! Challenge* do that in abundance. What was interesting to hear, was how although he exercised a lot during his 7-day challenge, he didn't feel hungry or feel he was overworking his body. He was able to sustain a lot of exercise whilst having just three balanced *Super Blend* a day and, as you just read, he also intends to carry on with a couple of blends a day. This, once again, helps to hammer home the point that by seeing significant results in a short space of time, you're much more likely to want to continue on your road to better health and a leaner body. It also helps if you:

a) Like the blends
b) Feel satisfied after having them
c) Have less desire for junk foods and drinks at the end of the challenge

And you will undoubtedly put a big tick next to all of the above, by the end of your challenge.

JOANNE O

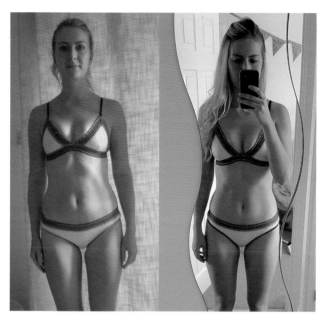

"I feel super happy with the results and I've actually got into my size 8 jeans with a little room around my belly, for the 1st time since having a baby!"

LOST 12lbs (5.4kg) IN 10 DAYS
LOST 3% BODY FAT
LOST 5cm OFF HIPS & THIGHS
GOT INTO **SIZE 8 JEANS**

"Thank you so much for letting me be a volunteer! After completing the Super Blend Me! 10-day challenge I feel super happy with the results and I've actually got into my size 8 jeans with a little room around my belly, for the 1st time since having a baby!! The first three days was a real struggle, I had a constant headache and was really tired. However by day 4 I felt a lot better and by Saturday it was just routine, I didn't even care that my friends were eating pizza and I was drinking my Super Blend! Although the last few days I have really craved a meal that I can actually chew. I was actually surprised how nice all the blends tasted and I will definitely be

carrying on to have them on a regular basis. I just want to say a massive thank you for helping me lose a chunk of my weight. I still have a little bit more I want to lose around my belly, but I know it will be a lot easier and quicker now I've been introduced to the Super Blend. So happy with the results, look forward to the launch of the book)."
Joanne O

MY THOUGHTS . . .

There are quite a few standouts here, but this one will resonate with many:

"I've actually got into my size 8 jeans with a little room around my belly for the 1st time since having a baby!!"

The fact she dropped 12lbs (5.5 kilos) and shaved 5cm off her hips and thighs (in just 10 days) will also resonate, but for many there's something about getting back into a pair of jeans that words can't often describe. The main point I want you to take away from Joanne's comments is that although the first three days were a struggle for her, by day four she was over the withdrawal hump, flying high and didn't even care that her friends were eating pizza as she was more than happy with her *Super Blend!*

It really is imperative you read the whole book, especially the *7 Rules and 7 Tips For Success*, as I cover the first three days and what to expect in depth. Not everyone struggles (as you have seen with the other examples so far) but it's good to know what withdrawal symptoms *may* occur, so you know how to mentally deal with them with ease.

STEVE V

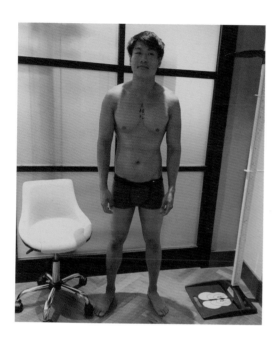

"I have more energy throughout the day, able to train more than once a day and still feel good."

LOST 5LBS (2.3KG) IN 10 DAYS
GAINED 3% MUSCLE
STOMACH FLATTER
LEANER AND TONED
SKIN CLEARER
SLEEPING BETTER

"I have completed the Super Blend Me! plan and I feel... Rebooted! My body feels lighter, cleaner and rejuvenated from the junk I was eating before. Skin is clear, stomach flatter, feel leaner, toned and less sluggish. I have more energy throughout the day, able to train more than once a day and still feel good. Feeling better, more positive and upbeat, not as stressed or unhappy. The urges for junk went away, it wasn't hard to resist junk after day 4 / 5. Sleeping quicker and waking up easier, without having to use the snooze button. This has to be my favourite Jason Vale plan – it makes you the most full and you only need a blender!"
Steve V

MY THOUGHTS . . .

Hard to know where to start with this one, as it appears he saw an improvement in just about every area, way beyond simply dropping weight and gaining energy. Yes, I appreciate that the main incentives for a great deal of the people reading this will be the weight loss and increased energy. But there is so, so much more you'll get out of this, as you will fully experience when you do it. Steve is sleeping better, his skin has improved, he feels less sluggish, he's not as stressed, he's happier, he's more positive and upbeat and, most importantly, his urges for junk have gone away. The reason I feel this is the most significant achievement is because it's long-term success that we should be aiming for, not a quick fix. It's all very well and good dropping some weight, but if your desire for junk is still there, you'll soon put it all back on the second you start munching on crap again. This is why his desire for junk being eliminated is so significant. At the end of his challenge he wanted to eat well and incorporate *Super Blends* into his lifestyle. So, even if you are the type of person who is jumping on the *Super Blend Me! Challenge* for a quick fix to get into that little black dress for the party next weekend, don't be surprised if by the end of it, you find yourself craving a salad!

I also really want to shout about the fact that, like so many others on the trial, Steve lost body fat and gained muscle mass. To be more specific, he actually gained 3% muscle mass, which is phenomenal, as he was pretty lean to start with. Clearly he was lifting weights too, but in order to build muscle you need to feed those muscles the right amino acids (building blocks for protein) post-workout, and because *Super Blend Me!* is rich in plant-based protein, it did the trick nicely!

The body cannot heal selectively; if you stop all the rubbish going into the body, whilst at the same time furnishing it with some of nature's finest natural fuel, everything will see some degree of improvement. So, if you are only doing this plan to lose weight, don't be surprised if your skin improves, your eyes start to sparkle and your hair starts to shine. Don't also be surprised if genuine lifestyle -related health issues start to improve, either. The body wants to heal and when you give it the time, space and right nutritional tools to do so, it will always do what it can.

NICOLE C

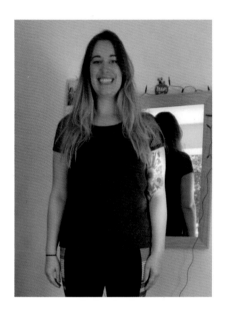

"I have lost 18lbs altogether, dropped two dress sizes and lost pretty much an inch from everywhere!"

LOST 18LBS (8.2KG) IN 14 DAYS
BODY FAT **DOWN 2%**
DROPPED 2 DRESS SIZES

"I have just completed the 14-day blend challenge and I have lost a total of . . . 18lbs!!! I feel light, accomplished, super proud, super healthy and ready to rock my wedding dress. I feel amazing. I have lost 18lbs altogether, dropped two dress sizes and lost pretty much an inch from everywhere! I can't wait to wear my wedding dress and feel confident, glowy and great!" **Nicol C**

MY THOUGHTS . . .

Nicol had her wedding coming up, which meant the *Super Blend Me!* trial came at the perfect time. However, even she couldn't have predicted just how good her results would be. She dropped a massive 18lbs in just 14 days and, in her own words, she is "ready to rock her wedding dress". I just hope she hadn't already had the final fitting for it, because having dropped two dress sizes it would have needed to have been taken in a notch or five! However, I'm guessing that having to take your wedding dress in just before the big day can't be the worst problem for a 'bride to be' to have!

HILARY K

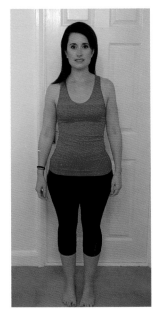 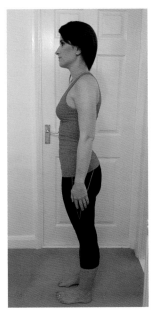

DROPPED 10LBS IN 7 DAYS!

"I feel amazing – it's rebooted my 'feel good' factor, my eyes are brighter, hair shinier, I feel slimmer & leaner. Bouncing around with so much energy."

MY THOUGHTS . . .

Hilary was actually checking in with me via Twitter as she tested the 7-day *Super Blend Me! Challenge*, so I know how much exercise she was doing alongside it. This is one of the many beauties of this pure blend plant-protein-based plan, you don't have to ease off your usual exercise routine to maintain your energy. Hilary's weight loss result for someone who was already in pretty good shape, is remarkable – 10lbs in just 7 days! However, it's the intangible results that I love the most: brighter eyes, shinier hair, more energy and the return of her 'feel good factor'. These results, although not exactly scientific, are still incredibly real and the most common improvements people report.

BECKY C

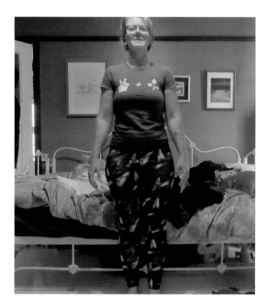

"...diabetes responded very well to the blends – I needed less insulin as my insulin sensitivity improved."

DIABETES **IMPROVED**
LOST 2.8 INCHES OVERALL
NO MORE ACHES & **PAINS**
FITNESS IMPROVED DRAMATICALLY

"I feel fantastic. More energy, more positive and happy, I am more motivated and feel lighter and cleaner. I have no aches and pains anymore. I have more energy to get through the day, and complete my exercise. I'm motivated, and look forward to exercising, whereas previously I was struggling with motivation and a desire to do anything active! I felt confident exercising with the blends, I had enough energy to do so. My diabetes responded very well to the blends – I needed less insulin as my insulin sensitivity improved. On average my insulin intake was about 12 units per day as opposed to 31 units previously. My insulin sensitivity has improved as a result of the programme and I feel it has provided some time for my body to have a break from my diabetes and readjust after a period of not taking sufficient care of myself. It will act as a catalyst to continue with positive eating and lifestyle habits." **Becky C**

MY THOUGHTS . . .

There are many headlines here, but for me the standouts are where she states "my diabetes responded very well to the blends...I needed less insulin as my insulin sensitivity improved", and "no more aches and pains". The reason why I see these as standouts is because, once again, *Super Blend Me!* isn't simply about dropping some weight – although that's always nice – it's about how it can improve the many, many areas of your overall health. When we chose people for the trial, I wanted to specifically test it on someone with diabetes. We have a crippling diabetes crisis and anything which can go in any way to helping reduce this must be a good thing. She also had the usual positive improvements from her *Super Blend Me! Challenge* – more energy, increased positivity, feeling more motivated, lighter, cleaner, plus no more aches and pains, and all this gave her the positive momentum to want to carry on to a healthy way of life. Or, in her own words . . .

"It will act as a catalyst to continue with positive eating and lifestyle habits"

SO, CONVINCED YET?
ITCHING TO START?
DON'T!

...WELL, NOT YET!
READ THE REST OF
THE BOOK FIRST

*Personally, I don't know how you could possibly
read these results and **not** be convinced.*

Remember, this is just a handful of results from those who took part in the trial, and I'm confident by the time you read this book thousands more from across the world will have achieved the same, if not better, results. I also don't know how you could possibly read and not only be convinced of the results this plan gets, but itching to try a *Super Blend Me! Challenge* on for size. Maybe you are, and can't wait to get cracking, but first I just need you to hang fire and heed this very important piece of advice – read the rest of the book first. Well, not all of it, you should wait to read the *Life After Super Blend Me!* (page 219) section until the final day of your *Super Blend Me! Challenge*. Let me repeat that, as it's extremely important you read the areas of the book at the right time:

READ:
LIFE AFTER SUPER BLEND ME!
on the final day of your *Super Blend Me! Challenge*

The remaining sections you **must** read, however, before you start the plan, are the *7 Rules For Success*, the *7 Tips For Success* and the entire Q & A. The Q & A in particular, will help to answer any unanswered questions you may have before you start, and will also be a great 'go to' throughout your challenge. I really would love to hear how you get on, so please drop me an email with the results of your *Super Blend Me! Challenge* to *results@superblendme.com* and / or post on my social media channels:

JuiceMasterJasonVale   JasonVale   JuiceMasterLtd   JuiceMaster

Pictures speak a thousand words, so please also try to include these where possible as your results will undoubtedly help to inspire others from all over the world.

Right, you have more reading to do, so it just remains for me to say:

GOOD LUCK, STAY FOCUSED,
DO WHAT IT TAKES

THE PLAN
SUPER BLEND ME!

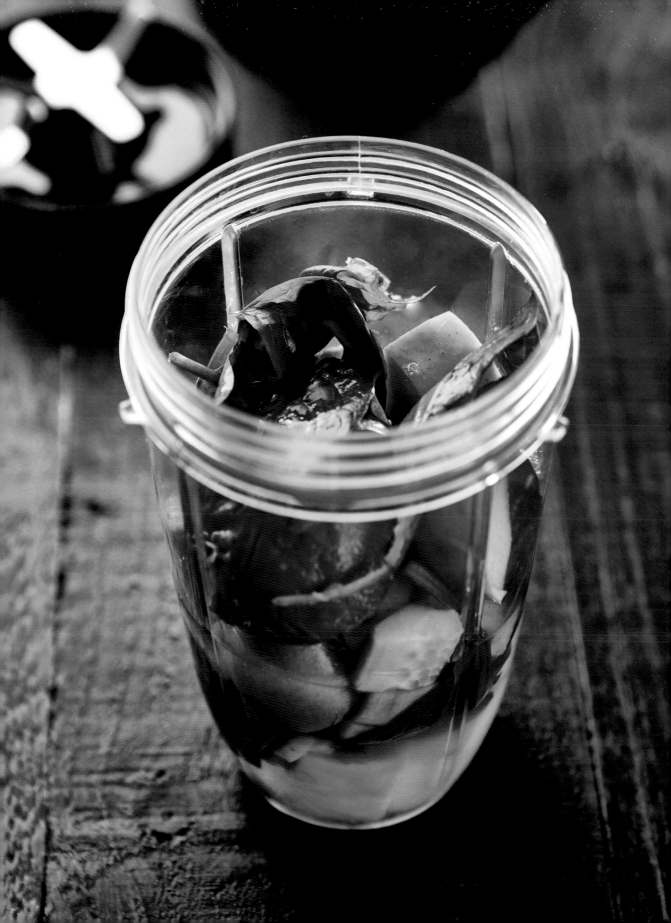

7
RULES FOR
SUCCESS

RULE 1

PICK YOUR OWN SUPER BLEND ME! CHALLENGE & STICK TO IT!

...AND ENJOY GETTING BACK INTO THOSE JEANS!

Super Blend Me! has been specifically designed with *everyone* in mind and you are free to pick from either a 7, 10, 14 or 21-day challenge. The minimum challenge, in order to see and feel tangible results, is 7 days and the maximum, depending on your personal situation, is pretty much open-ended. If you are in good shape, fairly fit and have only a few pounds to lose, then a 7-day challenge is probably what you need. However, if you are suffering with morbid obesity and many debilitating health issues, then a 21-day challenge should be the *minimum* you want to do. *Super Blend Me!* has been thought through nutritionally and can be continued for as long as a person needs to do it. Although some people, especially in the medical profession, will say that is something they would never recommend, I personally wouldn't hesitate in encouraging it if someone is morbidly obese and has a plethora of health issues. It's odd that many doctors wouldn't hesitate in recommending weight loss surgery to such an overweight person, but feel living on *Super Blends* for a significant period of time is potentially dangerous! Yes, it's abnormal to live on nothing but liquid nutrition, but it's also abnormal to be 400lbs in weight with a multitude of health issues. Sometimes we need to do something abnormal to counter the abnormalities we have created.

The point is, we are all unique and all have different health, body and fitness needs / goals, so it's important that you pick the plan that works for you. What I will say is, if you are someone who has anything up to 10-14lbs to drop, then you will see significant results in a 10-day *Super Blend Me! Challenge.* Clearly, I don't want to over-promise and under-deliver, but I can safely say that if you

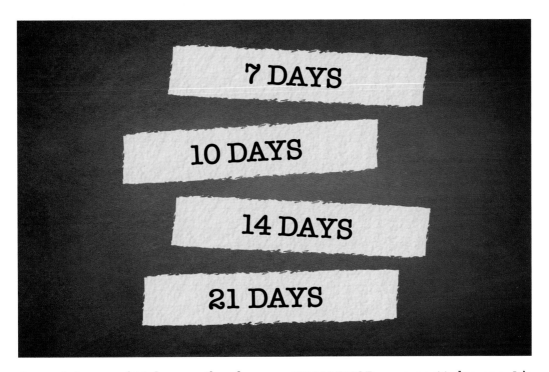

do a minimum of 10 days on the plan, you will see a very noticeable change in your body shape, health and energy levels – as already demonstrated with the *Super Blend Me!* test group.

If you are a couple of stone (28lbs) overweight (or more), and frequently feel tired and sluggish, then I would highly recommend the 21-day challenge. As mentioned, I personally tested this length of challenge, and I can honestly say I have rarely felt better. Whatever duration of challenge you pick – commit and stick to it! Don't pick the 21-day challenge and then justify bailing come day eleven, because you feel a bit better than you did. A 21-day challenge is just that, a **TWENTY-ONE-DAY**

CHALLENGE – not an 11-day one. It's easy to come up with excuses, but if you want to experience the incredible results a 21-day challenge can bring, make sure you do whatever it takes to complete it. Also, don't just pick a 7-day challenge if you know you have quite a bit of weight to lose and / or you need significant change, just because it's shorter and seemingly more doable – raise the game and do the length of challenge you know you need. Once again, the vast majority of people who have a little bit of weight to drop, or want to get shredded in a short space of time, tend to go for the 10-day challenge. Not only do you get amazing results, but you only sacrifice one weekend without using your teeth!

RULE 2

DRINK YOUR SUPER BLENDS IN THE TIME FRAMES LAID OUT, BUT LEAVE AT LEAST FOUR HOURS BETWEEN THEM

There are three *Super Blends* (SBs) a day, and I have set specific time frames for when they should be consumed. These are laid out in the plan itself, but worth repeating and explaining here:

Super Blend 1	**8am - 11am**
Super Blend 2	**1pm - 4pm**
Super Blend 3	**6pm - 9pm**

Your first *SB* (*Super Blend*) should be consumed anytime between 8am and 11am, your second, between 1pm and 4pm with the last one between 6pm and 9pm. Although you can have your SB at any time within those time frames, there **must** be *at least* four hours between finishing one blend and consuming the next one. For example, if you finish drinking your first *SB* at 11am, **do not** have your next *SB* until *at least* 3pm. The reason for the *minimum* four-hour rule is to prevent

you from consuming too much in too short a period of time. For instance, you wouldn't want to have your first blend at 11am and then your second, say two hours later; that would make for a very long day with only one blend remaining!

You are free to leave a five or even six-hour gap between *SBs*, providing you consume each one in the time frames laid out. Clearly, if you have your first one at 8am then you'll have to wait five hours before you hit the next time frame, which is cool because it still meets the 'minimum time between SBs rule.

When I did my challenge, the times I had my *SBs* changed all the time and were often governed by how hungry I felt. My own rough timings were:

SB1 @10am / **SB2** @3pm / **SB3** @7.30pm

When looking at timings between your *SBs*, you need to allow for the drinking time, too. Some blends may take a little while to drink (well, they *should* – see *Rule 3*) and so I didn't usually finish my 10am blend until around 10.30am, which is why my second *SB* wasn't until around 2:30 – four hours after I had *finished* my first one. So, if you have your first blend at 9am, once you've take into account the 30 minutes on average drinking time, you shouldn't have your second blend until 1.30pm, not 1pm – make sense?

Clearly you may choose to do things differently to make it fit around your life, but the time frames I chose worked for me. In addition to the three *Super Blends* each day, you of course have the option of two *Hunger SOSs* (see *Rule 4*). If you are having a five or six-hour gap between *SBs* and you start feeling like your sugar levels are dropping, you can always use a *Hunger SOS* then. If you work nights, simply adjust the time frames to suit.

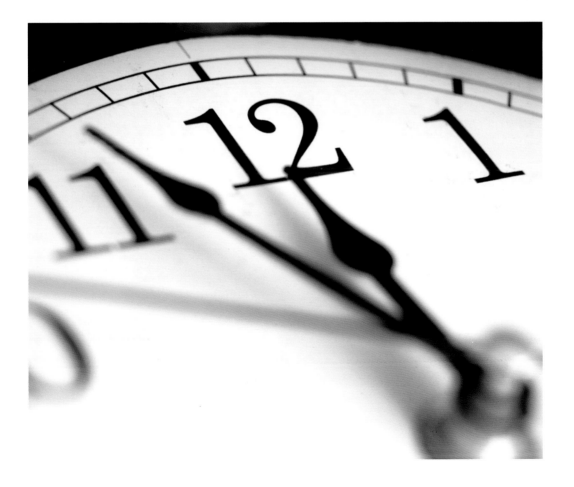

RULE 3

DRINK YOUR SUPER BLENDS SLOWLY

You should never drink anything you couldn't comfortably eat in the same time frame. I refer to this earlier in the book, and it's the *biggest* mistake people make when blending. You need to drink your blends *slowly* (think of taking your time with a fine wine) in order to allow enough time for comfortable digestion. It should take between 10–30 minutes to drink each SB, depending on the thickness and content of the blend.

DO NOT DOWN A BLEND IN A MINUTE FLAT!

Not only will you miss the wonderful flavours, but chances are you'll also get stomach cramps – so you have been warned! I personally take around 15–30 minutes per blend, as I like to savour the flavours and clearly want to avoid stomach problems; I advise you to do the same. Some of the blends are incredibly filling, which means you may not drink every blend in the one sitting (especially from day four onwards, after the *withdrawal hungers* have subsided). This happened to me a few times, and all I would do is drink half, pour the rest into a flask and pop it in the fridge for later. Another key rule while I am here:

ONLY DRINK YOUR BLENDS UNTIL SATISFIED

Like when eating, you should only drink your blends until you're *nicely satisfied* – not bloated. Just because all of the ingredients are good, it doesn't mean you can't have too much of a good thing. Your body only requires a certain amount of nutrition for your needs and is smart enough to tell you when it's had enough. Do not allow your mind to override your body. It comes as a surprise to many when, after the 72-hour withdrawal period, they start feeling much fuller for longer and, at times, either can't finish a blend or don't even feel like the blend at all. The reason for this is largely down to the body being *genuinely* fed. Many people are overfed and undernourished due to a lack of genuine nutrition in their diet. It is not about the *quantity* going in, but rather the *quality*. The old saying of 'less is more' is never more apt than when talking about the right nutrition going into the body. The irony is, that the vast majority of overweight and obese people are suffering from a form of malnutrition. The body will do whatever it can to turn junk food into usable fuel, but it will always need and continue craving the right nutrients for optimum health, by sending signals to the brain – aka, hunger. The problem is, junk food high in white refined sugar and refined fats is designed by BIG FOOD to be addictive, which creates additional, false hungers and the often-uncontrollable need for more. When you are feeding your body what it *actually* needs and eliminate the nutritionally empty, addictive and *additional hunger* causing junk foods, you start feeling genuinely satisfied and fuller for longer. This often comes as an unexpected but nice surprise to many, who expect to feel constantly hungry throughout their *Super Blend Me!* experience.

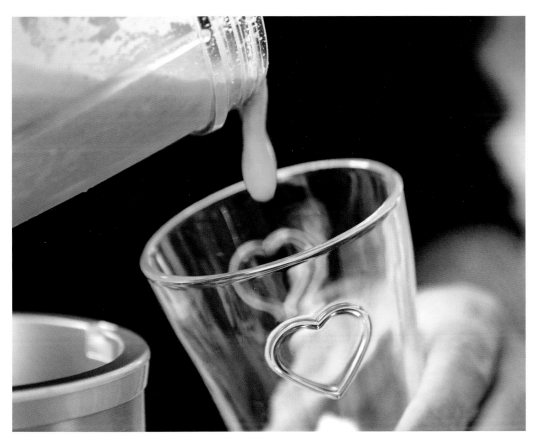

So, the key is to listen to your body and don't try to force-feed yourself the blends. If you're feeling full halfway through, pop the rest in a flask / bottle and drink later. Your body can only give you the signal of being genuinely satisfied if you drink your blends slowly, as instructed. This gives enough time for your body to send feelings of satisfaction to the brain.

One of the reasons I developed this plan was due to people blending the wrong things, in the wrong way. Not only blending things which don't belong in a blender and blending way too much insoluble fibre in a single blend, but also drinking their blends far too quickly and force-feeding themselves an entire blend because they think it means more goodness going in. Just because a blend is in liquid form, don't make the mistake of thinking what you are consuming is a drink – it's a *meal*, just in a glass! You may find, come the end of the day, that you haven't consumed all of your blends in their entirety, but don't worry. There were many times when I didn't consume all of my blends or even feel the need for a *Hunger SOS,* but providing you feel okay, it's okay! As long as you make a point of listening to your body and adhere to the 'only consume until nicely satisfied' rule, you'll be fine. I also kept to the rule of drinking my blends slowly, which gave my stomach time to send the signals to my brain when I'd had enough. I would then put the rest in the fridge to drink later, but more often than not, I didn't need to.

We are all different shapes and sizes and we all require different amounts of energy each day, so it's important to follow the rules and listen to your body. There are some who will have all of their blends and their *Hunger SOSs,* whilst there will be others who just won't be able to consume all of their blends and therefore have zero *Hunger SOSs* – both are perfectly fine. If you follow these rules, then you'll have great success on your *Super Blend Me! Challenge*; if you don't, you won't!

RULE 4

MAXIMUM OF TWO HUNGER SOSs A DAY

A *Hunger SOS* is a little something extra that you are allowed in addition to your blends, in the event of a genuine hunger emergency. You are allowed two per day on the *Super Blend Me!* plan and a cheeky *Hunger SOS* can often be the difference between success and failure. However, you should only use them when the need arises. A *Hunger SOS* can come into play if you miss a *SB* for some reason, you need something whilst out and about, in between blends or if you feel you will bail from the challenge completely, unless you can use your teeth. Your *Hunger SOS* can be one of the following:

1. **A piece of fruit.** Most go for either a banana, an apple, some melon or a medium avocado, cut in half, with a bit of cracked black pepper and a squeeze of fresh lemon juice (it even comes in its own bowl!).

2. **A natural energy bar.** Watch out for the false 'healthy headline' label tricks, such as *Natural* and *Fat-Free,* and always read the label. Most of the energy bars lining the shelves of supermarkets and advertised as 'healthy' contain shedloads of refined sugar, refined fats and artificial sweeteners – so be vigilant. Years ago, I couldn't find a good quality energy bar, so I produced my own. Luckily these days there are a number of genuinely good ones on the market, so you have plenty of choice. You're looking for a natural, good quality energy bar with no added nasties, so just make sure you do your homework first. I am biased clearly, but whenever I needed a cheeky extra something in between blends, I went for one of my *Juice SOS* bars (previously called *Juice In A Bar*) as they are full of nutrition and I know that everything in them is good. This bar, when first launched, won the *Best New Food Product of The Year* award – so I'm not alone in vouching for its quality!

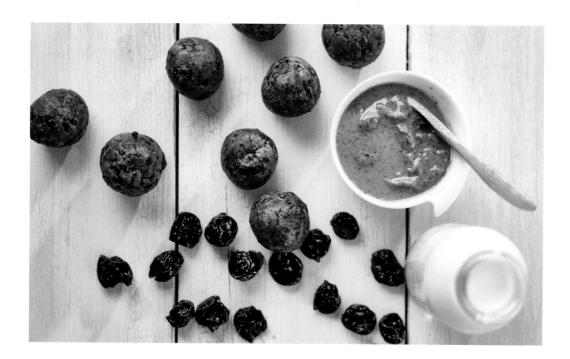

3. A homemade energy ball. I have included some cool energy ball recipes at the back of the book that you are going to love. You can easily make a batch of these, leave in the fridge and enjoy as and when needed. You can buy similar energy balls in most supermarkets now, but as they are so stupidly easy to make at home and way more cost-effective, if you have time – make your own.

Not everyone feels the need to ever use a *Hunger SOS* during their challenge as they really are designed to have as and when you *need* them. However, those who are blasting it in the gym or who don't have that much weight to lose and just want to clean up, may well feel the need to take advantage of both *Hunger SOSs* every day, for the entire challenge. If this is you, make sure you space them nicely between the blends. Personally, when I did 21 days, I was usually okay and had no need for a *Hunger SOS*, despite also doing 21 miles a day on the spinning bike. Having said that, when I did have my *Juice SOS* bar, it was usually in the evening, around 8 or 9pm, and I'd have it with a very large cup of peppermint tea. Incidentally, if you don't use your *Hunger SOS* for say three days, this doesn't mean on day four you can have all six in addition to the two for that day – **THIS IS NOT A ROLLOVER!**

RULE 5

USE COMMON SENSE WHEN EXERCISING DURING THE CHALLENGE

When it comes to exercise, it is vital you listen to your body. During the first 72 hours, most will experience some degree of withdrawal and in turn a slight or significant drop in energy. I spoke about this earlier in the book, but it's important you don't just blindly blast it in the gym if you are feeling at all shaky or weak. For most this doesn't happen, but if it happens to you, it's nothing to worry about, you just need to be intelligent and ease off until your energy returns (usually by day 4). The reason I bring this up is because when I did the plan, I was also doing 21 miles a day on a spinning bike. On day 2 I was in quite a bad way when I got off the bike. I was shaking, had to lie down and it took around 15 minutes and plenty of water before I was back to normal. I had pushed myself way too hard and didn't listen to my body. I wish to make this clear; I believe this would have happened anyway, even if I hadn't been on the plan. I was trying to beat my time and

simply pushed too hard. The good news is, by the end of the week and still on plan, I managed to beat my time – so it was clear that all I needed to do was pace myself. However, from week 2 I decided to break my exercise up. Rather than doing 21 miles straight on the spinning bike, I would do 10.5 miles in the morning and 10.5 miles after work. By breaking the exercise in half, I added two more positives:

1. **Less adrenal fatigue**
2. **Burned more calories**

A study on exercise and calorie-burn showed that if you only had 50 mins a day for exercise, but split it into two 25-minute workouts, you would burn an extra 400 calories. The study was done on cycling, but all relatively intensive exercise creates something called *after-burn*. After-burn does what it says on the tin, and means you *continue* to burn calories *after* you have finished exercising. If you

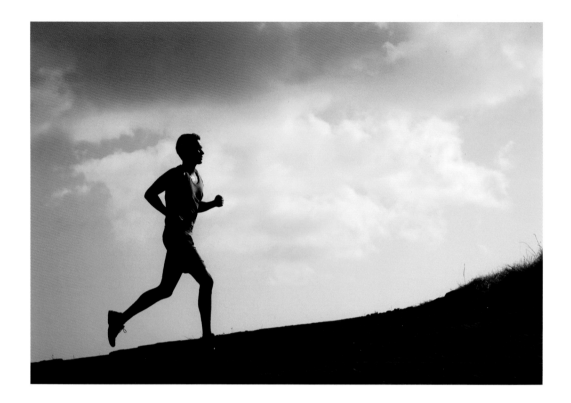

only have an hour to spare each day, splitting it into two 30-minute sessions will make it far more effective.

To be clear, you don't have to do intensive, or indeed any, exercise in order for *Super Blend Me!* to be successful. The reason I bring this up is because there will be many people who exercise on a daily basis, who will be attracted to this plan, largely because it's rich in plant proteins, good fats and the right carbohydrates. However, this doesn't mean you can't achieve incredible results if you only do light exercise (yoga, walking, etc.) or leave exercise out completely. You will be consuming nothing but perfectly balanced *Super Blends* for a *minimum* of 7 days, whilst eliminating all rubbish foods as well as alcohol, so you can't fail to drop some weight (if you need to) and feel a whole lot better than you did before you started. However, if you do (like most) want to step up the exercise – **USE YOUR COMMON SENSE AND LISTEN TO YOUR BODY.**

RULE 6

DON'T FREAK OUT IF YOUR SUPER BLEND IS SLIGHTLY OVER THE CALORIE COUNT!

If you have the new NutriBullet Balance *(smart bullet)*, you'll see that as well as being a fantastic blender, it also has the ability to work out the calorie count of your blend. It's as accurate as this type of technology allows, but it can never be 100% for many reasons. The key is not to get obsessed with the calorie side of life, and relax in the knowledge that the *Super Blend Me! Challenge* – providing you follow it to the letter – works!

Smart technology in products like the NutriBullet Balance can be a double-edged sword. It's been developed to let people know how many calories and how much protein, fat and carbohydrates are in the blends they make. This makes it a wonderful tool to help ensure you don't go overboard on excess calories, when making your own blends. However, it can also cause some people to become unhealthily obsessed with numbers! The good news is, the boys and girls over at NutriBullet HQ have decided to incorporate all of my *Super Blend* recipes into their new technology. It means when you open the NutriBullet Balance app, there will be a *Super Blend Me!* button so you'll not only have utter consistency with all the recipes, but they'll be no need to weigh or measure anything either. I think this is the best part about this new blender, you pop an ingredient in and it 'pings' at you when you've reached the required amount for the recipe (I know!) It will also tell you how many calories are in each one, but please don't get bogged down with the numbers. I have done all the work for you when it comes to the nutrition in *Super Blend Me!* – so just trust in the plan.

However, the vast majority of people will be using a non smart blender when doing the *Super Blend Me! Challenge*. If that's you, then you won't have any calorie numbers to look at, which won't be a bad thing here.

It's also worth pointing out that the body doesn't absorb all of the calories we consume. The percentage of calories absorbed will depend on what the food is. For example, we only actually absorb around 70% of the calories in certain nuts, like almonds. This means a 100-calorie serving of almonds in the kitchen is actually only a 70-calorie serving once in the body. Then you have to take into account that all of us will absorb calories differently. People with a higher proportion of Firmicutes bacteria absorb an average of 150 calories more than those with a higher proportion of Bacteroidetes (don't worry, you don't need to know what these are!). On top of that, you need to factor in someone's unique metabolism, which clearly affects the rate at which calories are burned. This is why these set, blanket guidelines for how many calories an average man and an average woman should consume are massively flawed. As a man, the guideline states that I need 2,500 calories a day, just to tick over for an average working day. However, if I were to consume 2,500 calories a day, without any exercise, I'd soon be as big as a house again. Whereas a good friend of mine can easily consume well over 2,500 calories a day, not exercise and nothing happens to his weight. Every decade your metabolism slows by about 10% too, so at almost 50, I need a lot less to help me 'tick over' than I did 20 years ago.

Calories have their place, and can be a wonderful tool when used correctly, as a *rough* overall guide, not as an exact science. For your reference, each blend in this *Super Blend Me! Challenge* is roughly 350 calories. This means just over 1000 calories a day, which may not sound like much, but please understand that it's the *quality* of the calories you are having, not the *quantity*. Having done the challenge myself, I can say with complete confidence that, in terms of calories and nutrition, you'll be good to go. I burnt over 800 calories a day on the spinning bike whilst on the three blends. This means, according to the calories *in* = calories *out* theory, I was 'ticking over' on just 250 calories a day – 10 times *less* than the suggested guidelines. This simply doesn't add up, because my energy levels were pretty consistent throughout, and I was even writing a book, running my company and doing talks at the same time. I am aware that just over 1,000 calories a day doesn't seem like much, but it's only for a short period of time, and, once you allow for that cheeky extra bit of nut butter whilst making your blend (trust me, you will) an extra banana here and there, and perhaps the odd *Hunger SOS*, it will be more like 1,200 calories a day. You will know what feels right for you, but please don't get obsessed with calories, trust in your instincts and the plan I have provided.

RULE 7

LET COMMON SENSE PREVAIL

Although *Super Blend Me!* works as it is for the vast majority of people, some may need to adjust it slightly. If you're a 7ft tall professional rugby player, for example, you'd be forgiven for having an extra blend or a couple more *Hunger SOSs* a day. However, if you're not a professional athlete with a trim body fat percentage, then you might not be so easily forgiven.

Please also don't make the mistake of immediately linking *everything* to the fact you're on the *Super Blend Me!* plan. You wouldn't normally analyse your day / week in terms of what you are eating. However, the second you're on a 'detox', everything that happens is *because* of the 'detox'. Get a cold on day 3 – it's the 'detox'. Feeling tired at 4pm on day 5 – it's the 'detox'. Get a pimple on day 8 – it's the 'detox'. Having a bad hair day – it's the 'detox'. You have a bad day at work on day 9 – it's the 'detox'. I think you get the point. Life has its ups and downs whether you're on just *Super Blends* or not, and it's important to understand that.

As with everything, when on *Super Blend Me!* be sensible and let common sense prevail at all times.

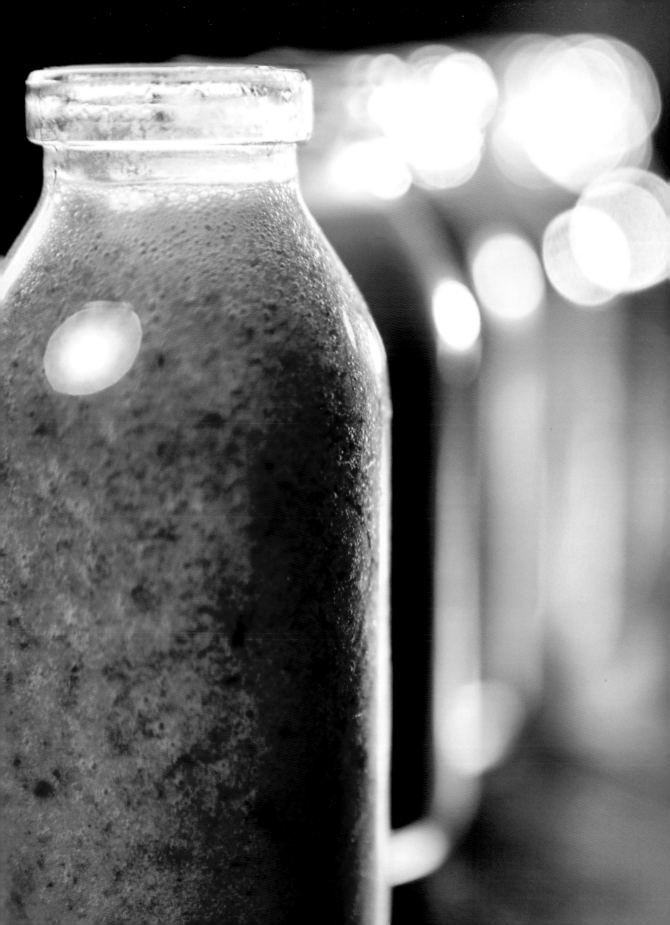

7

TIPS FOR
SUCCESS

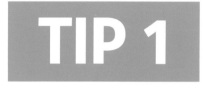

TIP 1

GET YOUR MIND FULLY PREPARED!

Do not underestimate the extremely important role your mind will play throughout your *Super Blend Me! Challenge*. How you manage your thoughts before, and throughout, will make the difference between whether you succeed or fail. You can get all the prep right in terms of shopping, the right blender, clearing your social calendar, etc., but if you don't manage your thoughts correctly, you'll struggle and / or fail. I have covered the correct way to manage your mindset earlier in the book (*The Main Withdrawal Is In The Mind*, page 25) so if you haven't already read it, please make a point of doing so. It isn't a simple case of positive thinking or whether you are strong-willed or not, it's about the *correct* way of thinking. If you manage your mental approach to the challenge, and think in a way that serves you, you'll smash it. If you don't, you'll constantly struggle and, ironically, the stronger willed you are the *quicker* you'll cave in. This is not a misprint and I urge you to read that part of this book (if you haven't already) to really get to grips with mastering my *Freedom Thinking Technique* rather than just *positive* thinking. If you have already read it, I strongly believe that repetition is the mother of all skill, but rather than just re-reading the chapter, you may want to check out the app, which features a whole load of videos that complement the book as well as a couple of exclusive SOS videos, which you can access anytime, anywhere. I would also make a point of watching my *Super Juice Me!* documentary before you start. Although *Super **Juice** Me!* is not *Super Blend Me!* the documentary is incredibly inspirational and will give you even more impetus to do your challenge.

TIP 2

LET YOUR FREEZER & CUPBOARD BECOME YOUR BEST FRIENDS!

The main benefits *Super **Blend** Me!* has over its *Super **Juice** Me!* rival, are *speed* and *convenience*. It's faster because, unlike a juicer, a blender literally takes seconds to clean, and more convenient, because you can use frozen produce when blending. Avocados, berries, spinach, kale, bananas and even ginger can all be blended from frozen, but not juiced. You may think that fresh is always best, but not only is that not always the case, there's also many circumstances in which frozen is actually *better* than what is deemed as *fresh*. Many fruits in supermarkets masquerading as fresh often have less nutrients than their frozen friends. This is because they are picked before they are ripe, and therefore given less time to develop a full range of vitamins, minerals and antioxidants. Fruits and vegetables can spend weeks in transit before getting to a distribution centre. Some, like apples and pears, can be stored for a whole year under controlled conditions before being sold. Fruits and vegetables that are picked when fully ripe and frozen immediately retain their nutrient value. Unlike applying heat, cold *preserves* life (if in doubt, think IVF and frozen embryos) which is why you really don't need to worry if you're using frozen produce for *Super Blend Me!*

What I would advise though, is when it comes to greens and leaves such as mint, basil, kale, broccoli, cucumber and spinach – go fresh. Yes, you can buy things like frozen spinach and kale, which can be extremely convenient as spinach goes off pretty fast, but most frozen spinach has also been blanched before it's frozen. Blanching involves placing the produce in boiling water for a short time, which kills any harmful bacteria and prevents loss of flavour, colour and texture. The problem is, it also causes the loss of water-soluble nutrients such as B vitamins and vitamin C. Please note that this doesn't apply to frozen fruits, as they don't go through the blanching process.

I used frozen fruits throughout my *Super Blend Me! Challenge*, as not only is it simply more convenient to do so, but they are often more nutritious for reasons already mentioned. If you wish to use frozen veggies like kale, spinach and broccoli but want to avoid the blanching, simply freeze them from fresh yourself. This means you have full control over the quality of the spinach, etc. you are buying. You may, of course, choose to do this with your fruits too, especially if you grow your own, or have a cool farm nearby (it's always good to support local if you can). When you add frozen fruits to a *Super Blend*, they add a wonderful creaminess (especially things like banana and pineapple) whilst also negating the need to add ice. If you find some really good *ripe* avocados, buy as many as you can and freeze them. Clearly don't freeze them as they are, cut them in half, remove the large seed and scoop out the flesh. Once you have done this, simply add to a freezer bag or freezer-friendly locking container and pop in the freezer. While I am here, the same goes for bananas; don't freeze them with the skin on – they don't peel well frozen! So, peel them first and cut into halves before freezing. You can even freeze things like pineapple – simply peel and dice. It's worth clearing some space in your freezer and freezing as much of this stuff as you can before you start the plan, as it will help to make the process even easier! Most people shop for everything they are going to need for week one on the Sunday (as most start on a Monday) so if you shop early in the day, you can spend a lot of Sunday in *freezer prep* mode. So, if you want to make it super-easy and convenient, frozen is definitely the way to go. However, if you choose to buy and refrigerate your produce, the only things you have to really have to keep an eye on are spinach, mint, basil and kale (spinach being perhaps the worst for fridge life).

As for the rest of the ingredients, all the milks and coconut water keep for a good few days in the fridge (even if you make your own almond milk you can store it for three days) and everything else you'll need can be stored in the cupboard. This is, without question, the quickest and most convenient plan I have ever devised, and it's almost impossible to come up with a reasonable excuse as to why you can't do it. I have tried to make sure there is as little waste as possible by repeating each of the main recipes twice throughout the week, and I have tried to repeat the main ingredients throughout, too. The good news is, because most of the ingredients are either frozen or cupboard items, if you do have anything left over it won't go off and therefore won't go to waste. I can guarantee you'll feel so good after the challenge that whatever you do have left

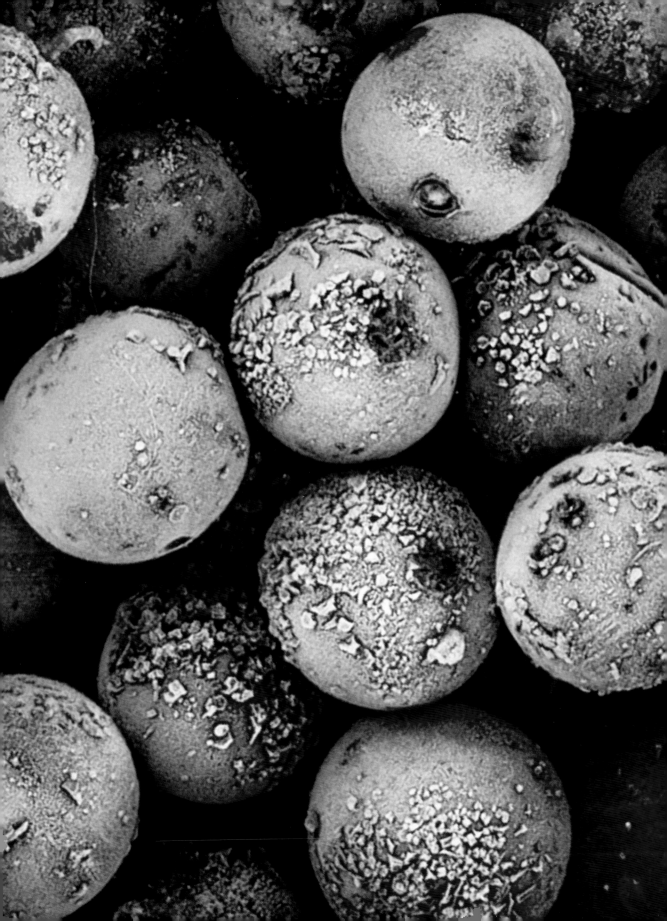

over will soon get used up, as I have no doubt that you'll be introducing *Super Blends* into your everyday life.

If you get prepared both in terms of organisation of your produce and getting into the correct thinking mode (see *Tip 1* page 76) you'll knock this challenge out of the park. If you have the *Super Blend Me!* app, it gets even easier. Not only do you have everything you could possibly need at the touch of a button, such as all the recipes and a plethora of videos, including two *SOS* videos that I have personally recorded to support you through any wobble moments, the *7 Tips & Rules for Success* and *Life After Super Blend Me!*, but it also has an auto-generating shopping list function. This means you can pick the amount of days you wish to shop for and it will work out a shopping list for you. There really is no excuse; just get as prepared as you can to give yourself the best possible chance of completing your *Super Blend Me! Challenge* to the letter. Before we move on to the next tip, here's a snippet from one of the people who took part in the *Super Blend Me!* test trial, which I feel demonstrates perfectly just how your freezer and the right prep can make life so much easier:

> "A very good plan... I thought I would feel lethargic and lacking in energy doing this plan as that's how I have felt previously doing diets. I had absolutely no lack of energy at any point and no headaches. Personally, I think asking somebody who works and has a busy life to make 3 drinks every single day, whilst keeping all the ingredients in and fresh is just a near impossible task...so I made Sunday my day of making 21 drinks for the next 7 days and numbering the bottles and freezing them all fresh, it worked a treat. I also used a bigger blender than the one you provided which allowed me to make 2–3 500ml drinks at a time (again much easier)" **Jimmy G**

I personally disagree that it's impossible for someone who works and is busy to make three blends a day, but Jimmy found a way to make it easier for himself and on Sundays he made all the blends and simply froze them. If you feel that even that's too much effort, it's worth mentioning you can now get the 10-day *Super Blend Me!* plan sent direct to your door through *juicemasterdelivered.com*. The main message of *Tip 2* though, is to make your freezer and cupboard your best buds.

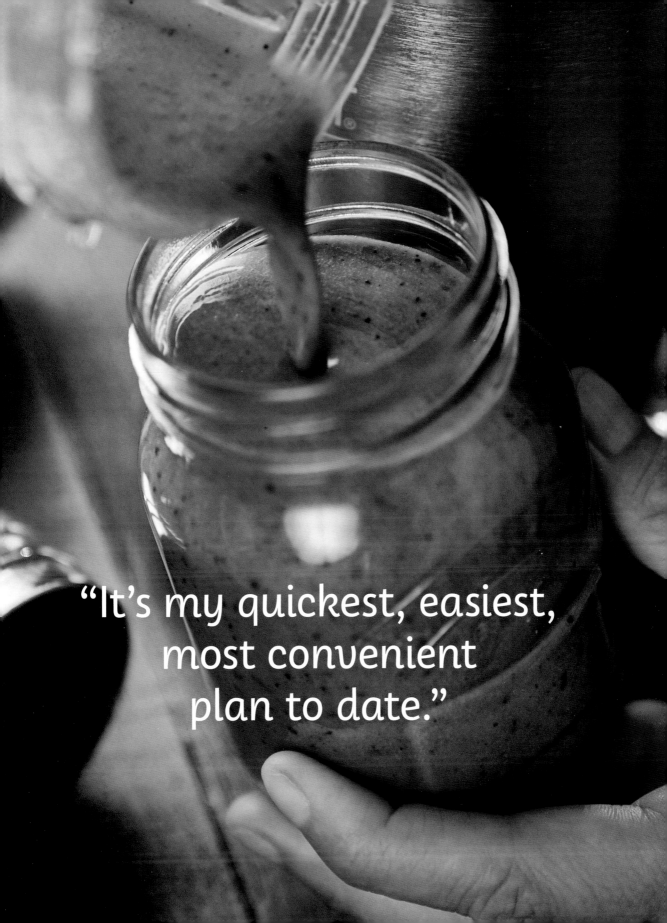

"It's my quickest, easiest,
most convenient
plan to date."

TIP 3

GET THE RIGHT KIT!

They say it's a bad workman who blames their tools, but if your tools aren't up to scratch, you're never going to get the best results. Not all blenders are built the same and if yours isn't up to much, your blends may not turn out as they should. The main players in the blending world at the time of writing this are the NutriBullet and the NutriBullet Balance, which is why I started the book talking about the NutriBullet phenomenon. However, they're not the only players. There are many really good blenders on the market; the key is to get the right one for *you*.

For most, a bullet-type blender is perfect. Not only are they the best-selling blenders in the world in terms of how they perform, but also for convenience, as the blending cup you make the blends in doubles up as your drinking cup too. These bullet-type blenders usually come with different lids, usually a sealed storage lid and a flip-top drinking lid. They also tend to come with a couple of cups, so if you're doing the plan with someone else, you're good to go. As already mentioned, the leader in this field is NutriBullet and when it comes to making this plan even easier, the new NutriBullet Balance is the perfect piece of kit for this plan as they've integrated the recipes. Having said that, the only slight frustration with bullet type blenders is that if there's more than one of you doing it, you'll have to make the recipe twice, as each cup only holds a single serving. This brings me onto the other type of blender, which is more suitable if a large number of you are doing at the plan at the same time. Large upright blenders are extremely common, but not all make the grade. Currently, the best on the market are the Vitamix and Blendtec, but neither are cheap! There are other good upright blenders, but you need to do your homework so I advise checking out the reviews first.

The only other piece of kit you'll need is a good flask. There will be times when you will want to blend and go and your bullet cup may not be enough, especially if you are taking a couple of blends with you for breakfast and lunch. You're looking for a flask that is airtight, can hold the right amount (there's approx. 500ml per blend) can easily fit ice cubes in (as not all can) and looks cool. Ok, so I have added the final feature because I use our *It's A Juice Thin* flasks, which are uber cool – but clearly a cool looking flask is not a prerequisite. Oh, and if you are planning on freezing your blends, make sure you check that the flask you are using is freezer-friendly. If you have the right blender and right storage containers, it will make your challenge so much easier.

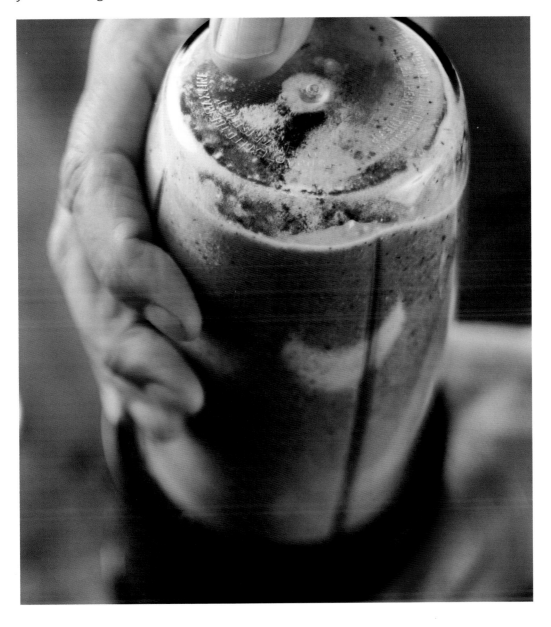

TIP 4

CHOOSE THE PATH OF LEAST RESISTANCE

Before starting the challenge, pick the path of *least* resistance but don't not pick a path because of *some* resistance. What I mean is, there will never be the perfect time to do a challenge of this nature, but some times are clearly better than others. You will always have something in the diary that coincides with you doing *Super Blend Me!* It could be a dinner party, wedding, weekend away, or just a lunch date you had locked in. If you are doing the 7 or 10-day *Super Blend Me! Challenge* then it will be easier to clear some time, but if you are doing the full 21 days, you'll just have to accept that it won't be *as easy* in terms of clearing diary commitments – but it's still completely doable. What I would say is, don't choose times which cross over your birthday or something like Christmas or Thanksgiving, there are plenty of other windows of time open to you without you having to deny yourself a decent holiday season or birthday. I also would try to avoid big social gatherings like weddings or parties, so if you know you have one coming up, you may wish to start your challenge afterwards. I would also tell those close to you what you are doing and, even if they don't agree with it for whatever reason, ask for their support while you're on the challenge. I'll cover the resistance you can encounter from others and how to deal with it in *Tip 5* (coming up next) but I would make a point of letting people know what you are doing so they can work around it. I realise that there will be some of you who will not only encounter resistance from others, but who may well still have to cook your family dinner whilst on the *Super Blend Me!* plan. Things like this, along with certain social commitments, may be unavoidable no matter what window you look for in your diary, but my tip is to check your diary before you start and choose the path of least resistance. There will always be some resistance, but don't use it as an excuse not to start.

TIP 5

DON'T LET OTHERS PUT YOU OFF WITH THEIR BS!

There are two reasons why you might get some crap from people for doing the *Super Blend Me! Challenge*:

1. Lack of, or just plain false knowledge about nutrition
2. Not wanting you to improve your house while theirs remains the same!

The problem with the subject of nutrition is that, due to the sheer volume of books and interest in the subject, everyone's an expert. There are probably more heated debates about nutrition, and what approach is best, than almost any other subject. Everyone has an opinion and many have very strong opinions that they feel everyone should hear. The good news is that by doing Super **Blend Me!** you won't get as much crap as those who do my Super **Juice Me!** plan, but chances are you'll still get *some* crap. This usually either comes from incredibly ill-informed people who don't have a full understanding of nutrition, or just from people who secretly know that it will work wonders, but don't want you to do it for fear it will work wonders for you (crazy I know!). It's like if you live next door to your best friend and you decide to give your house a cheeky makeover. By taking the time, effort and energy to improve your house you have now, inadvertently, made their house look worse. Now they have one of two choices to make their house look as good, if not better, than yours. They can either spend the time, effort and energy improving their house – as you've done – or they can blow your house up! Unfortunately, consciously or subconsciously, they tend to do the latter (I'm speaking metaphorically, of course!). I remember when I was a smoker and all of my friends smoked, too. The second I said I was giving up, they would do whatever they could to either prevent me from making the attempt or to try to tempt me back once I had stopped. They didn't do this because they were evil, but because *me* not smoking highlighted even more *their* inability to stop. It's the same with weight and health. If you and a friend are overweight and you tell them that you are about to embark on the big *Super Blend Me!* 21-day challeng – which will drastically change your weight, health and energy – chances are, they will do whatever they can to make sure you either don't start or don't finish. Again, they do this not out of genuine malice (although some do!) and often their behaviour is extremely subconscious, but nobody wants to be left behind. If you get slim, trim and healthy, it will highlight the fact they are not. So, if anyone gives you any BS for doing the challenge, know why they are doing it and don't let them put you off. Some, of course, aren't doing it out of any jealously or fear of you improving your 'house' (so to speak), but rather because they have a lack of understanding about nutrition. There are still some, we need to remember, who think you can't get calcium or protein unless you drink cow's milk or eat the cow itself. You may even think this yourself! This is why you need to put your nutritional needs in my hands, just for the duration of your personal *Super Blend Me! Challenge*, and see how you look and feel at the end. That is the only time at which to judge and have an informed opinion as to whether this works! It amazes me the number of people who have a strong, often negative opinion about my plans, yet have never actually done even one of them. I have personally tested all of my plans, including *Super Blend Me!,* which is why I can say with utter confidence you have zero to worry about on the nutrition front while you are doing it.

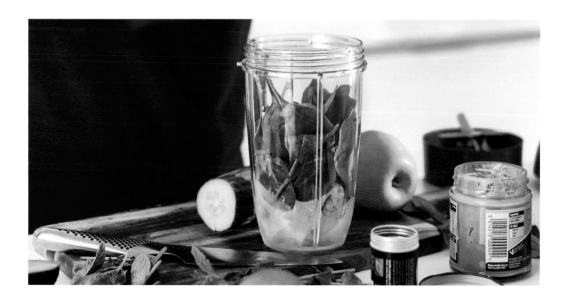

TIP 6

EMBRACE THE OPPORTUNITY TO FULLY INDULGE

One thing's for sure, when you're not cooking or going out as much, you have lot more time in your life. In order to gain even more from your *Super Blend Me! Challenge*, I advise embracing the opportunity to fully indulge. Many people make the mistake of thinking a challenge of this nature is all about deprivation, but on every level, nothing could be further from the truth. Firstly, as mentioned earlier, if you tap into the correct thinking, rather than indulging in the usual diet mentality of 'moping around for things you hope you won't actually have' – which is a form of utter insanity – you definitely won't feel deprived on the food front. Secondly, rather than feeling sorry for yourself and focusing on where you *can't* go and what you *can't* do during the challenge, why not really focus on the many opportunities for personal indulgence this challenge *can* bring? In today's extremely fast-paced and screen-led world, many of us rarely find time to fully nurture ourselves. You will be nurturing yourself nutritionally throughout your *Super Blend Me!* journey, but this is also the perfect time to nurture your mind and soul. You will find that your body, in the absence of false stimulants and the addition of wonderful nutrition, will naturally want to rest in order to repair and fully recharge. We often blindly stay awake because we feel it's too early to sleep, but if you are tired at 9pm, don't fight it, go to bed; get a full recharge on every level. Take this opportunity to run a bath, light some candles, maybe get some nice relaxing oils, relaxing music and a good book. If you're a member of a gym – especially if it's one with a pool, sauna, steam, etc. – spend the evening there. You can take your *Super Blend* in a flask, do your workout, and drink it in the sauna. It's also a good way to socialise on the challenge, as you won't be sitting there watching people drinking or having a nice meal! Many of these clubs have loungers and are open till around 10pm. The best part is that after around 8.30pm, most people have gone home (to have dinner!) which means you pretty much have the place to yourself. Take a book and have a mini spa break every night. The point is, embrace the extra time available and focus on all of things you *can* do, rather than what you feel you *can't*. I don't know your personal situation or what's available to you, but an early night, hot bath and a good read is usually open to most. It's nice to have an excuse to just stop. As well as a mind and body 'detox', it might also be worth, especially during your relaxed indulgent evenings, having a 'digital detox', too. The place where you'll see more food than anywhere else is on Instagram, so it might be worth skipping it. I would certainly avoid Twitter too, not because you may see lovely recipes, but because it's just too angry on there. You want to surround yourself with as much positivity as possible and Twitter is most certainly not the place for that. If you aren't a book person, then why not use this opportunity to indulge in some uplifting and educational documentaries and films, or download an audiobook?

Weekends, of course, are slightly different as you tend to have *a lot more* time on your hands and there's usually a lot more temptation, especially as a lot of people use junk food and alcohol as their wind down after a busy week. Once again, *embrace* the opportunity to do things you perhaps wouldn't usually do. Everything from spending full days at your gym with the pool, sauna and steam, to finding a beautiful walk in your area, or a gallery, maybe even a matinee theatre performance. There really is so much out there to do, you just need to take the time to open your eyes and see what's around. If you live in a major city there is *no excuse* as there are thousands of ways to fill your time. You may also find, after the first three days, that your mind becomes sharper too (it can happen in the absence of alcohol and junk, oddly!). So, perhaps this is the time to start that book you were going to write, or make plans for that new business you were going to start. The key is to not mope around or feel sorry for yourself, but rather really embrace the many, many opportunities to indulge that this challenge brings. This is not about deprivation but rather feeding your mind, body and soul exactly what it needs.

TIP 7

MIX IT UP IF YOU FEEL THE NEED

You will notice that I use just nine key *Super Blend* recipes throughout the first 7 days. You may also notice, if you are doing a 10, 14 or 21-day *Super Blend Me! Challenge*, that the same 7-day plan gets repeated. If you are doing longer than 7 days, you may feel the need to mix it up a little and introduce some of the other *Super Blend Me!* recipes. You are more than welcome to do this, providing you only use the recipes from the *Extra Recipes* section (page 139) as they are all *Super Blend Me!* ready. It is also important to include a green one, protein one and a fruit one each day and so the key is to swap like for like. So, if you're switching out a green one, make sure it's for another green one; a berry one should be replaced with, you got it, another berry-based recipe (I think you get the idea!). I have also included three *Special Guest Super Blends* as part of the plan, which appear every Friday, Saturday and Sunday, so there's no chance of getting bored. Especially as I've included four additional *Extra Special* recipes, so you can change things up a little if you wish. Having said that, chances are you won't want to mix it up and will simply use the *Extra Recipes* and *Extra Specials* at the back of the book, as general day-to-day *Super Blends*, after you have finished the plan. This is because, not only are the *Super Blends* on the plan perfect in terms of nutritional balance, but each recipe is only repeated a maximum of twice throughout a 7-day period. A little FYI, if you do choose to switch out one of the main plan recipes for one of the *Extra Recipes,* or one of the *Special Guests* for an *Extra Special*, you'll have to adjust your shopping accordingly (which is another reason why I like the app, as it conveniently works it all out for you). Personally, I kept to the plan as designed. I never got bored of the recipes because they're not repeated enough to get bored, and it was easier to shop for the plan 'as is'. Most of the ingredients also cross over and I designed it this way specifically, to reduce waste.

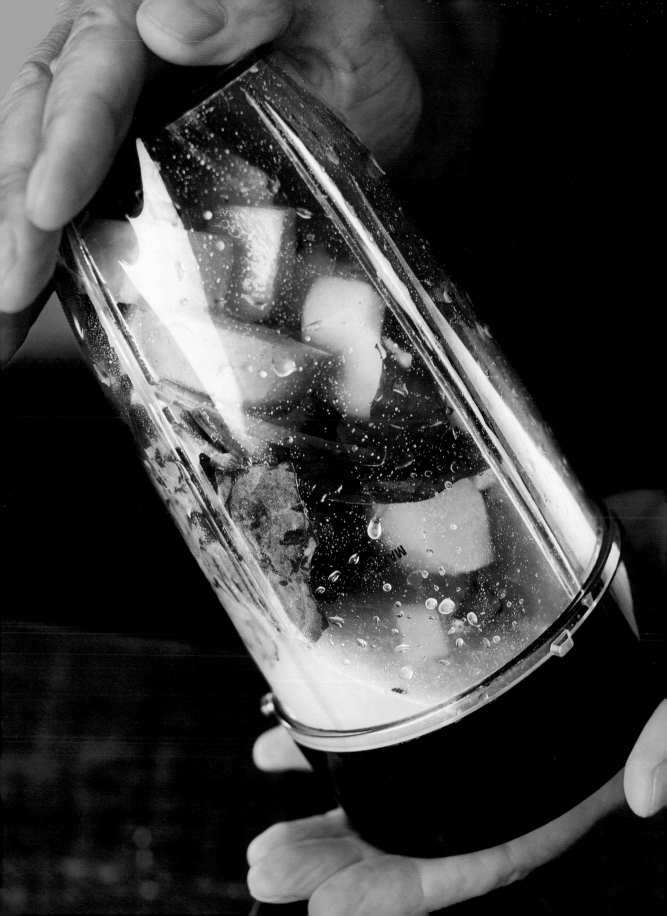

SUPER
BLEND
MASTERY
In 4 Easy Steps!

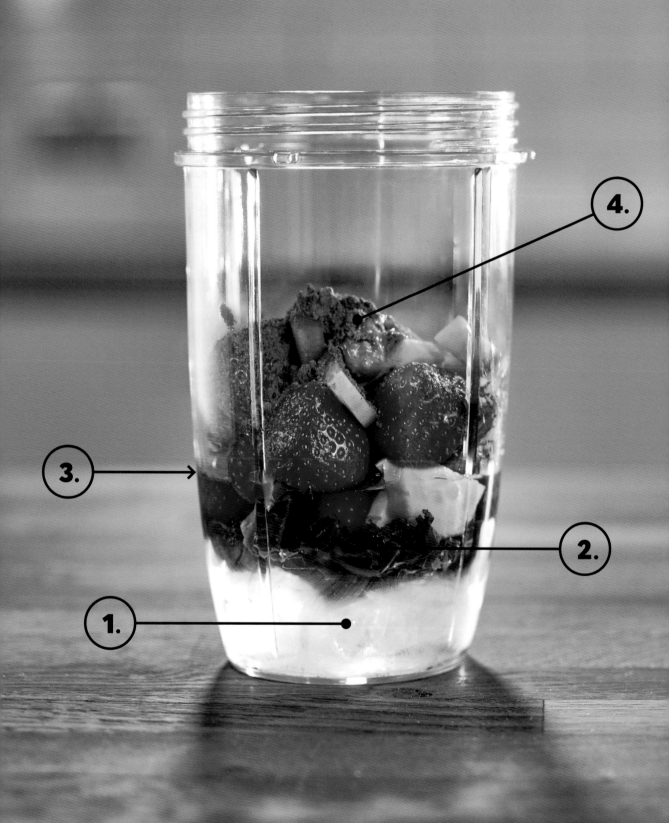

1. Keep It Cool

First thing to put into your blender when making your *Super Blends* is ice. The key to a good tasting blend is temperature, especially when veggies are involved. In addition to keeping your *Super Blends* deliciously cool I have also added ice as part of the overall liquid content; however, if you want to leave it out, you can, it just means you will just end up with a slightly thicker, warmer blend. If you are using frozen fruits then your Super Blend is already going to be cool, but a little extra ice won't hurt!

2. Keep It Healthy

Second thing to add to your blender are any fruits, veggies, leaves or seeds the recipe requires. Spinach, kale, cucumber, avocado, banana, mint, mango, berries, etc. all get added at this very important second stage, and it's where the core nutrition of the *Super Blend* lies.

3. Keep It Drinkable

Third thing to add to your blender is the liquid side of life. Unlike juicing, if you don't add liquid to the other ingredients in your blend, you'll be eating it rather than drinking it! In your *Super Blend Me! Challenge* you'll find just four key liquids – almond milk, coconut milk, coconut water and oat milk.

4. Keep it Super!

Last thing to add to your blender are any powders, pastes or butters that the recipe calls for. These are, in my opinion, the key ingredients that will transform your blend into a Super Blend. Firstly, when you add in rich, creamy nut butters such as almond or cashew, there is no question the taste and texture is transported from okay to true super status. Secondly, although fruits, veggies and leaves make up the core nutrition of your blend, the powders, pastes and butters also raise the nutritional game substantially. The optional *Super Blend Me!* powders – *Green*, *Berry* and *Protein* – is where you'll find ingredients like spirulina, wheatgrass, goji berries, etc.

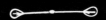

~ *Super Blend Me!* ~
7-DAY PLAN

~ *Super Blend Me!* ~
10-DAY PLAN

—∘———∘—

7-DAY PLAN × 1 . . . THEN REPEAT FIRST 3 DAYS

[1–7] + [1, 2, 3]

~ *Super Blend Me!* ~
14-DAY PLAN

—∘———∘—

7-DAY PLAN × 2

[1–7] + [1–7]

~ *Super Blend Me!* ~
21-DAY PLAN

—∘———∘—

7-DAY PLAN × 3

[1–7] + [1–7] + [1–7]

~ Let's Go Shopping ~
7 DAYS

PRODUCE	QUANTITY FOR 7 DAYS
Almond Butter	6 teaspoons
Cashew Butter	4 teaspoons
Coconut & Almond Butter	3 teaspoons
Tahini	3 teaspoons
Almond Milk	1000 ml
Oat Milk	1000 ml
Coconut milk (carton not tin)	1000 ml
Coconut Water	2150 ml
Yoghurt (your choice i.e. bio-live, vegan, coconut)	6 tablespoons
Cacao or Cocoa	2 heaped teaspoons
Sunflower Seeds	4 tablespoons
Oats	2 tablespoons
Medjool Dates	4
Mixed Berries	3 handfuls
Blueberries	4 handfuls
Pomegranate Seeds	3 tablespoons
Strawberries	3 handfuls
Raspberries	2 handfuls
Peas	2 tablespoons
Banana (small)	14
Avocado (medium)	2
Apple	1
Lime	4
Spinach	11 small handfuls
Kale	8 small handfuls
Mint	7 small handfuls
Pineapple	½
Cucumber	1
Protein Powder (Hemp / Pea)	100 grams
Ice	1 bag

~ Let's Go Shopping ~
10 / 14 / 21 DAYS

QUANTITY FOR 10 DAYS	QUANTITY FOR 14 DAYS	QUANTITY FOR 21 DAYS
9 teaspoons	12 teaspoons	18 teaspoons
6 teaspoons	8 teaspoons	12 teaspoons
4 teaspoons	6 teaspoons	9 teaspoons
5 teaspoons	6 teaspoons	9 teaspoons
1700 ml	2000 ml	3000 ml
1250 ml	2000 ml	3000 ml
1500 ml	2000 ml	3000 ml
2850 ml	4300 ml	6450 ml
8 tablespoons	12 tablespoons	18 tablespoons
2 heaped teaspoons	4 heaped teaspoons	6 heaped teaspoons
6 tablespoons	8 tablespoons	12 tablespoons
2 tablespoons	4 tablespoons	6 tablespoons
5	8	12
4 handfuls	6 handfuls	9 handfuls
6 handfuls	8 handfuls	12 handfuls
3 tablespoons	6 tablespoons	9 tablespoons
5 handfuls	6 handfuls	9 handfuls
3 handfuls	4 handfuls	6 handfuls
2 tablespoons	4 tablespoons	6 tablespoons
21	28	42
3	4	6
2	2	3
6	8	12
16 small handfuls	22 small handfuls	33 small handfuls
12 small handfuls	16 small handfuls	24 small handfuls
9 small handfuls	14 small handfuls	21 small handfuls
¾	1	1.5
1.5	2	3
160 grams	200 grams	300 grams
1½ bags	2 bags	3 bags

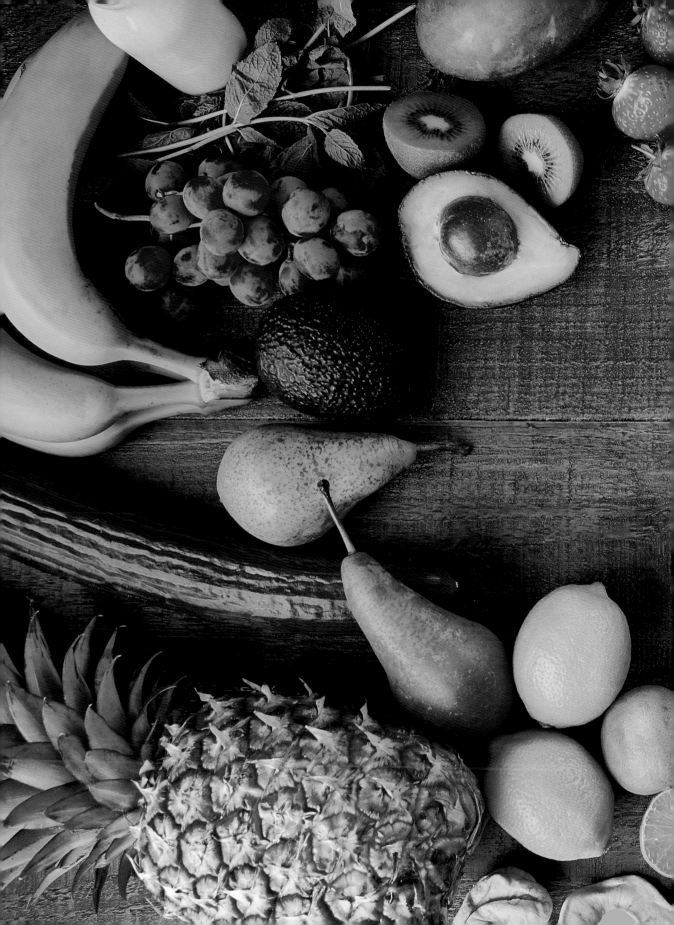

Super Blend
PLAN
RECIPES

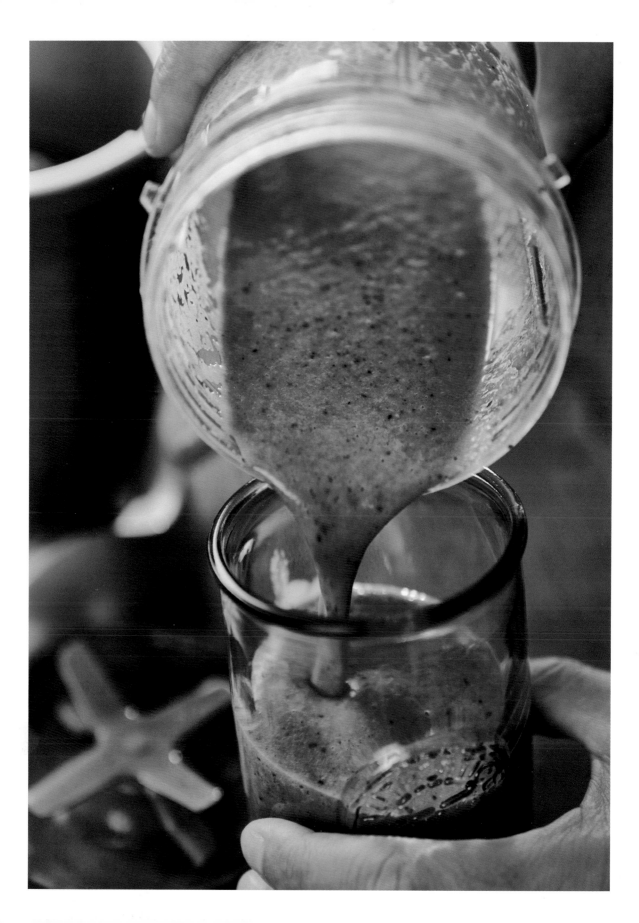

Blue 'n' Green Protein Queen

HOW TO DO IT!

Peel the cucumber and chop into small pieces. Add the ice to your blender. Scoop in the flesh of the avocado, followed by all other ingredients. Blend for 15 – 30 seconds.

Pea or hemp protein powder are also good alternatives.

INGREDIENTS:
Serves 1

Ice
1 small handful

Cucumber
2½ cm chunk or 1 small handful

Avocado (ripe)
¼

Spinach
1 small handful

Blueberries
1 handful

Fresh Mint Leaves
1 small handful

Oat Milk
250 ml

Almond Butter
2 teaspoons

Protein SBM! Powder*
1 tablespoon

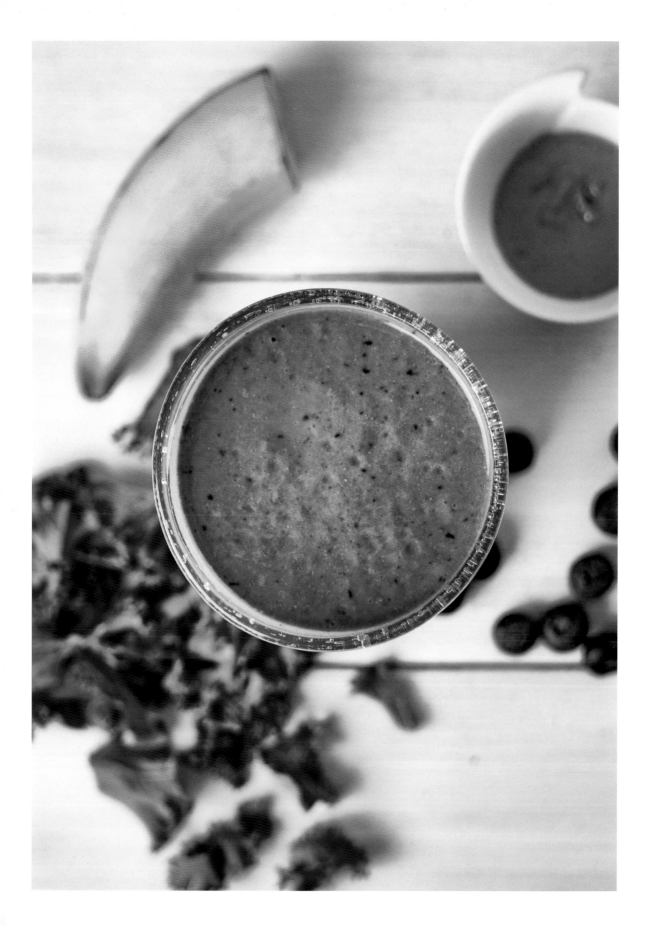

Blueberry Kale & Cashew Crunch

HOW TO DO IT!

Add the ice to your blender, followed by all other ingredients. Blend for 15 – 30 seconds.

INGREDIENTS:
Serves 1

Ice
1 small handful

Banana
1 small

Blueberries
1 handful

Kale
1 small handful

Sunflower Seeds
1 tablespoon

Coconut Milk (carton)
250 ml

Cashew Butter
1 teaspoon

Berry SBM! Powder (optional)
1 teaspoon

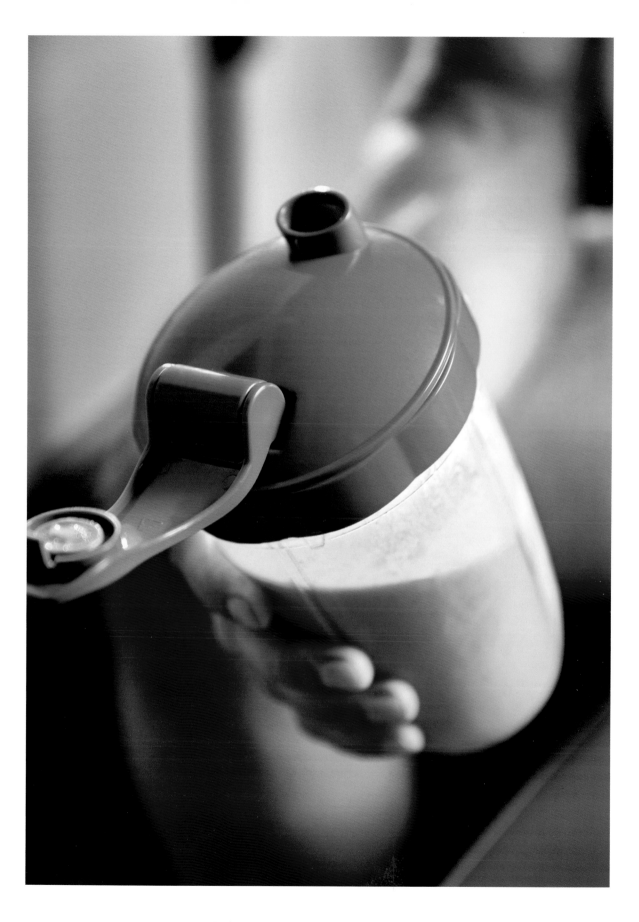

Creamy Nut Butter Protein Blast

HOW TO DO IT!

Remove the stone from the date. Add the ice to your blender, followed by all other ingredients. Blend for 15 – 30 seconds.

Pea or hemp protein powder are also good alternatives.

INGREDIENTS:
Serves 1

Ice
1 small handful

Medjool Dates
1

Banana
1 small

Almond Milk
300 ml

Almond Butter
1 teaspoon

Cashew Butter
1 teaspoon

Protein SBM! Powder*
1 tablespoon

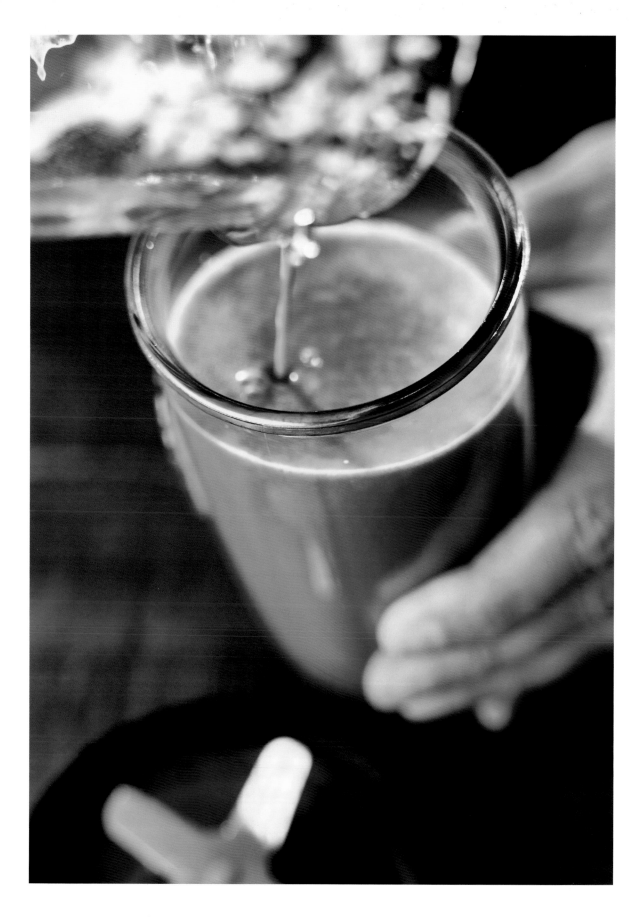

Minty Green
Super Blend

HOW TO DO IT!

Add the ice to your blender. Scoop in the flesh of the avocado, squeeze in the lime juice, followed by all other ingredients. Blend for 15 – 30 seconds.

INGREDIENTS:
Serves 1

Ice
1 small handful

Avocado (ripe)
¼ medium

Lime
1 (juice of)

Kale
1 small handful

Spinach
1 small handful

Banana
½ small

Fresh Mint Leaves
1 small handful

Coconut Milk (carton)
250 ml

Green SBM! Powder (optional)
1 teaspoon

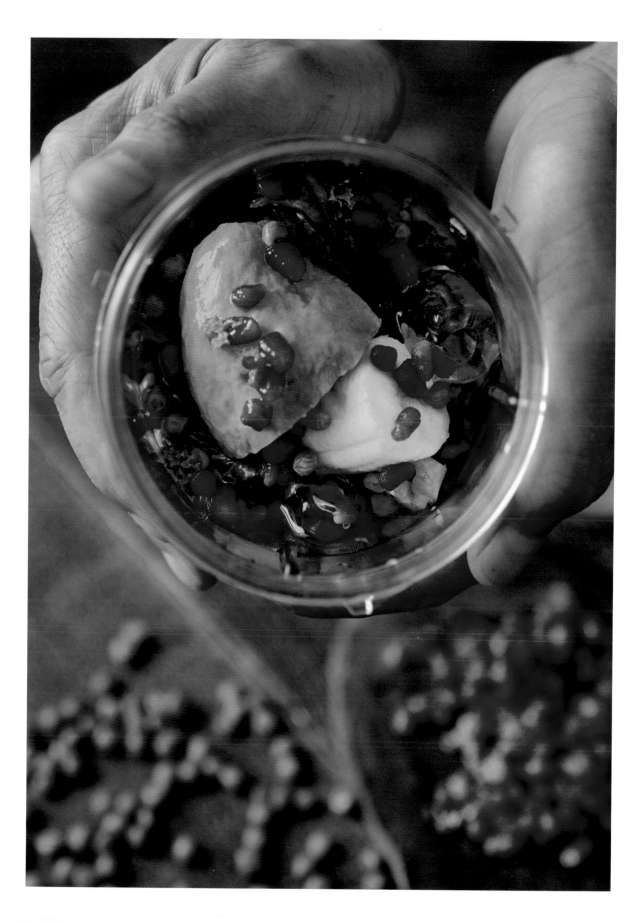

Pea 'n' Pom Avo Super Blend

HOW TO DO IT!

Add the ice to your blender. Scoop in the flesh of the avocado, followed by all other ingredients. Blend for 15 – 30 seconds.

INGREDIENTS:
Serves 1

Ice
1 small handful

Avocado (ripe)
¼

Banana
½ small

Spinach
1 small handful

Kale
1 small handful

Peas
1 tablespoon

Pomegranate Seeds
1 tablespoon

Fresh Mint Leaves
1 small handful

Coconut Water
250 ml

Green SBM! Powder (optional)
1 teaspoon

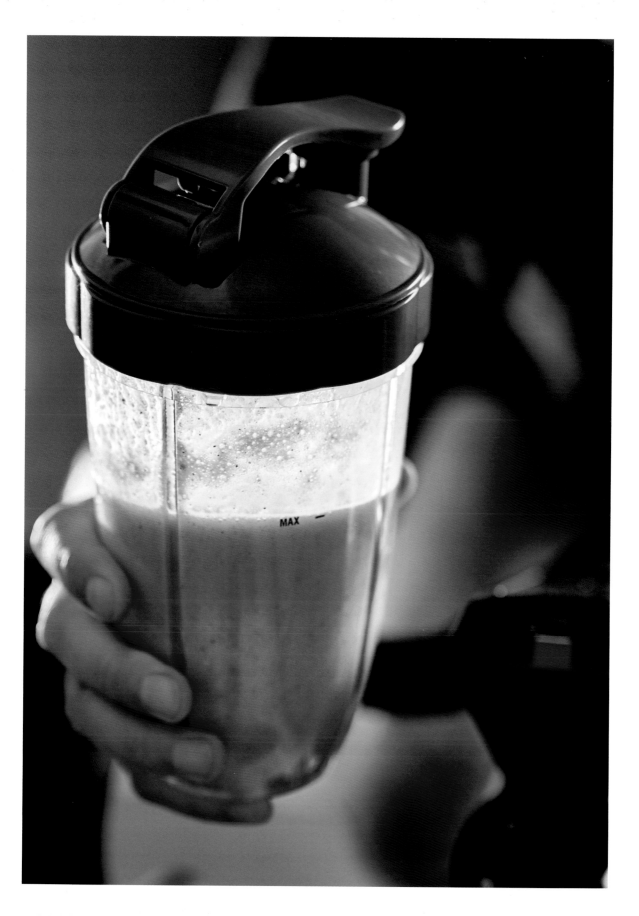

Raspberry Coconut Protein Shake

HOW TO DO IT!

Add the ice to your blender, followed by all other ingredients. Blend for 15 – 30 seconds.

*Bio-live, coconut or other alternative.

**Pea or hemp protein powder are also good alternatives.

INGREDIENTS:
Serves 1

Ice
1 small handful

Banana
1 small

Raspberries
1 handful

Coconut Water
250 ml

Yoghurt*
1 tablespoon

Coconut Almond Butter
1 teaspoon

Protein SBM! Powder**
1 tablespoon

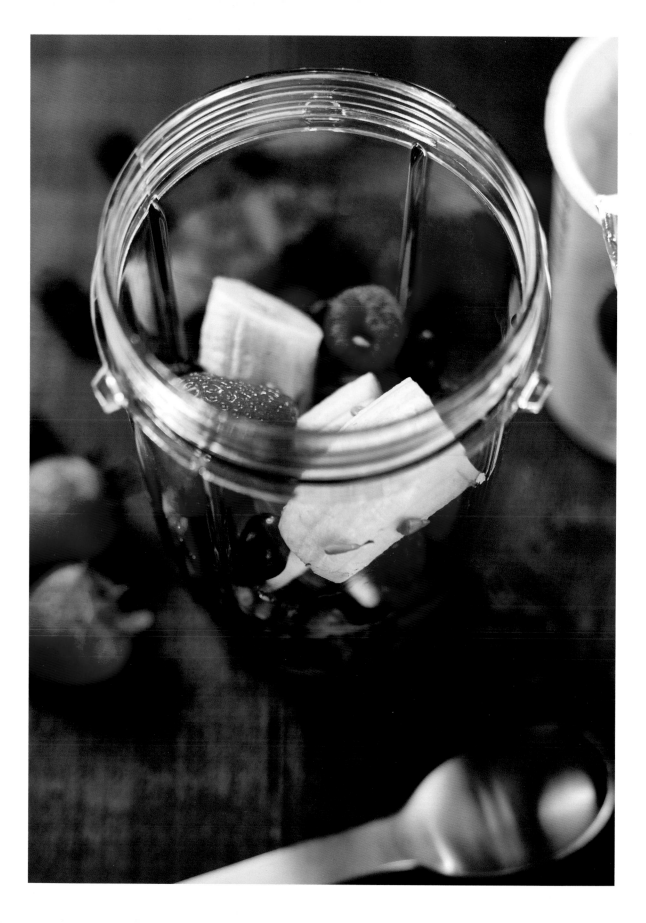

Super Berry Blast

HOW TO DO IT!

Add the ice to your blender, followed by all other ingredients. Blend for 15 – 30 seconds.

Bio-live, coconut or other alternative.

INGREDIENTS:
Serves 1

Ice
1 small handful

Mixed Berries
1 handful

Kale
1 handful

Banana
1 small

Sunflower Seeds
1 tablespoon

Coconut Water
250 ml

Yoghurt*
1 tablespoon

Berry SBM! Powder (optional)
1 teaspoon

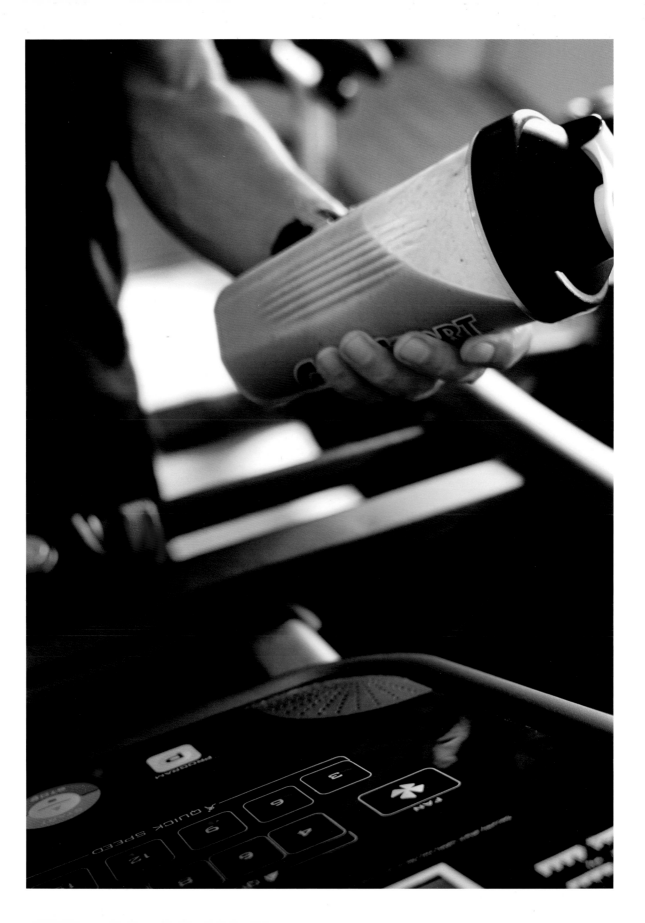

Tahini Protein
Berry Blast

HOW TO DO IT!

Peel the cucumber and chop into small pieces.
Remove the stalks from the strawberries.
Add the ice to your blender, followed by all
other ingredients. Blend for 15 – 30 seconds.

Pea or hemp protein powder are also good alternatives.

INGREDIENTS:
Serves 1

Ice
1 small handful

Cucumber
2½ cm chunk or 1 small handful

Strawberries
1 handful

Banana
1 small

Spinach
1 small handful

Almond Milk
200 ml

Tahini Paste
1 tablespoon

Protein SBM! Powder*
1 tablespoon

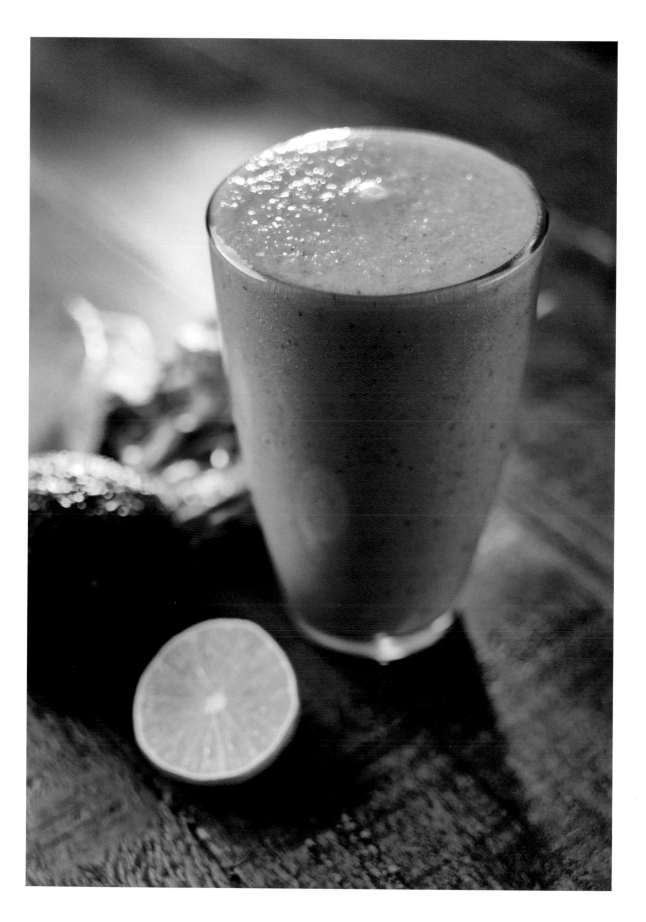

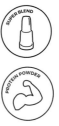

Turbo Charge
Super Blend

HOW TO DO IT!

Remove the core from the apple and chop.
Peel the pineapple and cucumber and chop
into small pieces. Add the ice to your blender,
scoop in the flesh of the avocado, squeeze
in the lime juice, followed by all other
ingredients. Blend for 15 – 30 seconds.

Pea or hemp protein powder are also good alternatives.

INGREDIENTS:
Serves 1

Ice
1 small handful

Apple
½

Pineapple
2½ cm slice or 1 handful

Cucumber
5 cm chunk or 1 handful

Avocado (ripe)
¼ medium

Lime
1 (juice of)

Spinach
1 handful

Coconut Water
200 ml

Protein SBM! Powder*
1 tablespoon

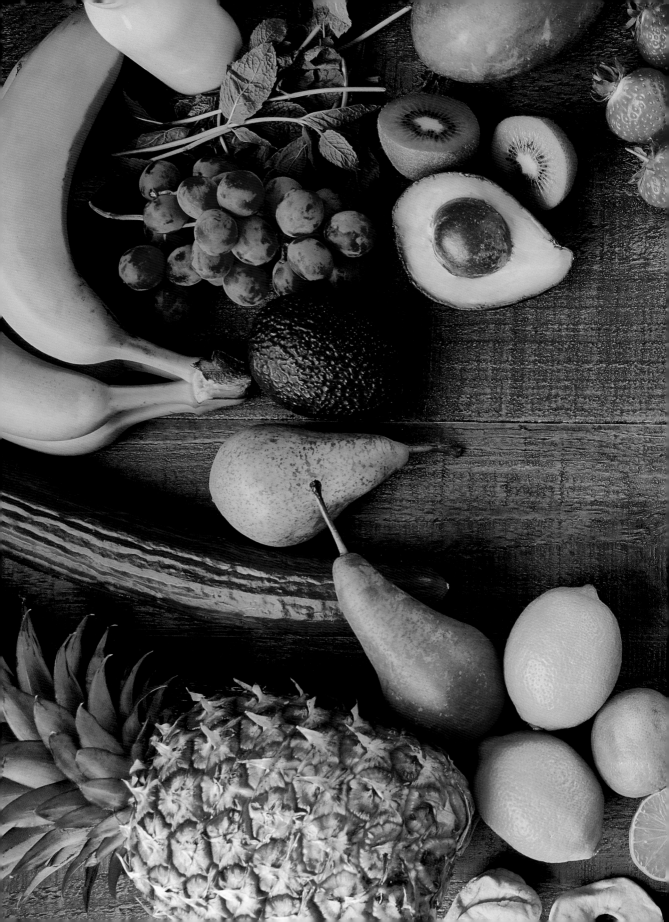

Special Guest
PLAN
RECIPES

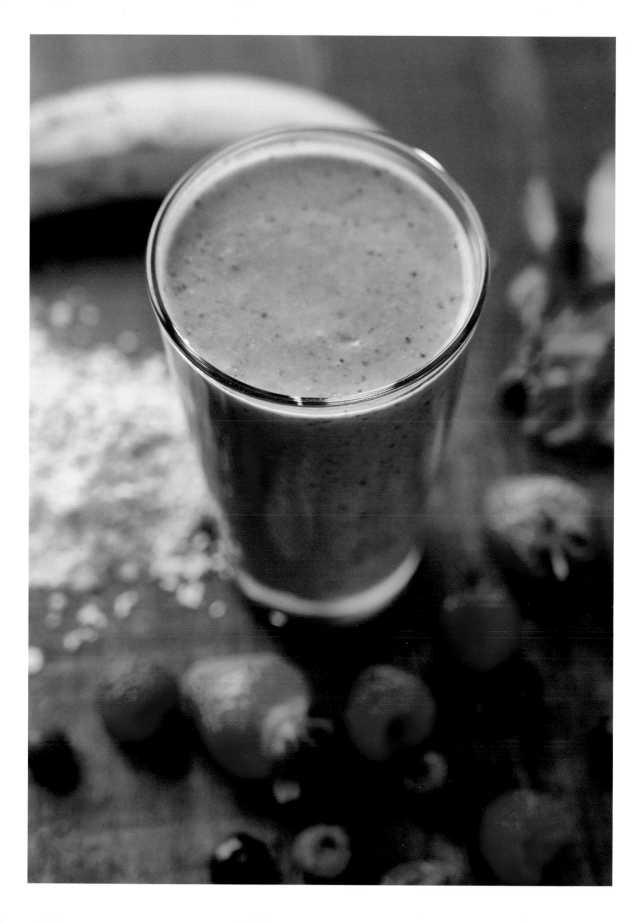

Brekkie
Super Blend

HOW TO DO IT!

Remove the stone from the date. Add the ice to your blender, followed by all other ingredients. Blend for 15 – 30 seconds.

Bio-live, coconut or other alternative.

INGREDIENTS:

Serves 1

Ice
1 small handful

Medjool Dates
1

Banana
1 small

Mixed Berries
1 handful

Spinach
1 small handful

Oats
2 tablespoons

Oat Milk
200 ml

Yoghurt*
1 tablespoon

Berry SBM! Powder (optional)
1 teaspoon

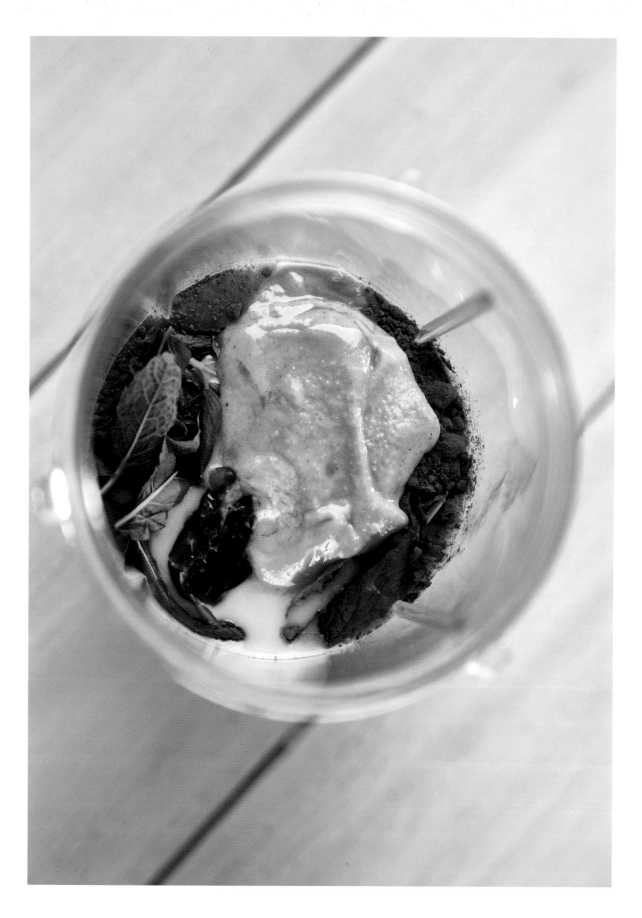

Mint-Choc Tahini Beaney

HOW TO DO IT!

Remove the stone from the date. Add the ice to your blender, followed by all other ingredients. Blend for 15 – 30 seconds.

INGREDIENTS:
Serves 1

Ice
1 small handful

Medjool Dates
1

Fresh Mint Leaves
1 small handful

Banana
1 small

Oat Milk
300 ml

Tahini Paste
1 tablespoon

Raw Cacao Powder
2 heaped teaspoons

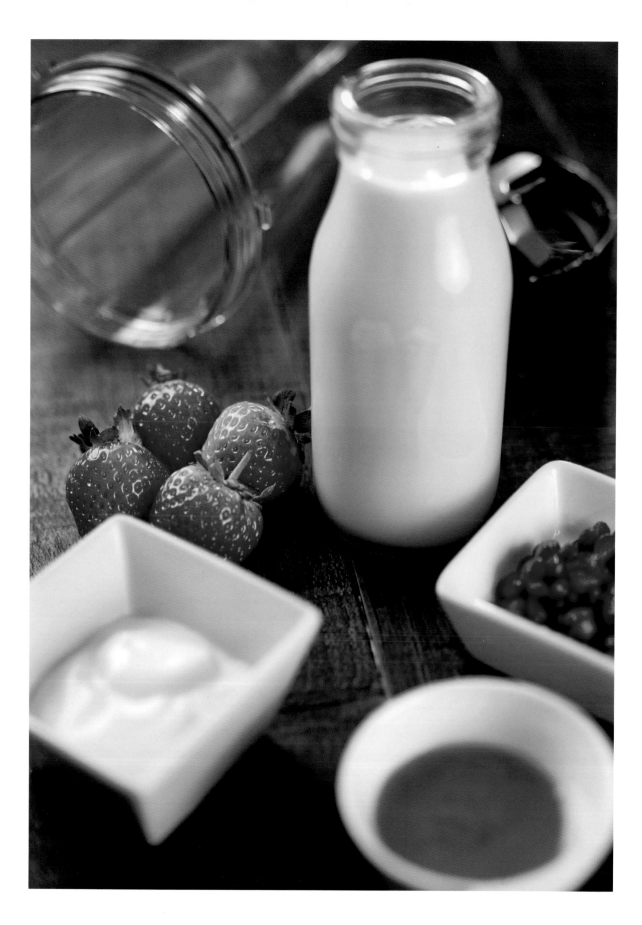

Strawberry Coconut Cream

HOW TO DO IT!

Remove the stalks from the strawberries. Add the ice to your blender, followed by all other ingredients. Blend for 15 – 30 seconds.

Bio-live, coconut or other alternative.

INGREDIENTS:
Serves 1

Ice
1 small handful

Strawberries
1 handful

Pomegranate Seeds
1 tablespoon

Coconut Water
250 ml

Yoghurt*
1 tablespoon

Coconut & Almond Butter
1 teaspoon

Berry SBM! Powder (optional)
1 teaspoon

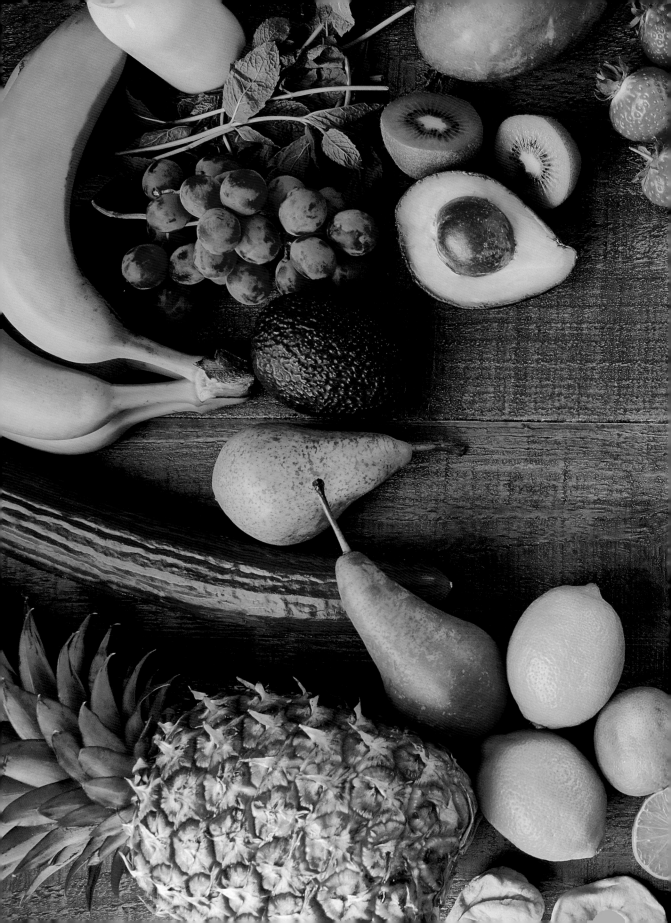

Extra
SPECIAL
GUESTS

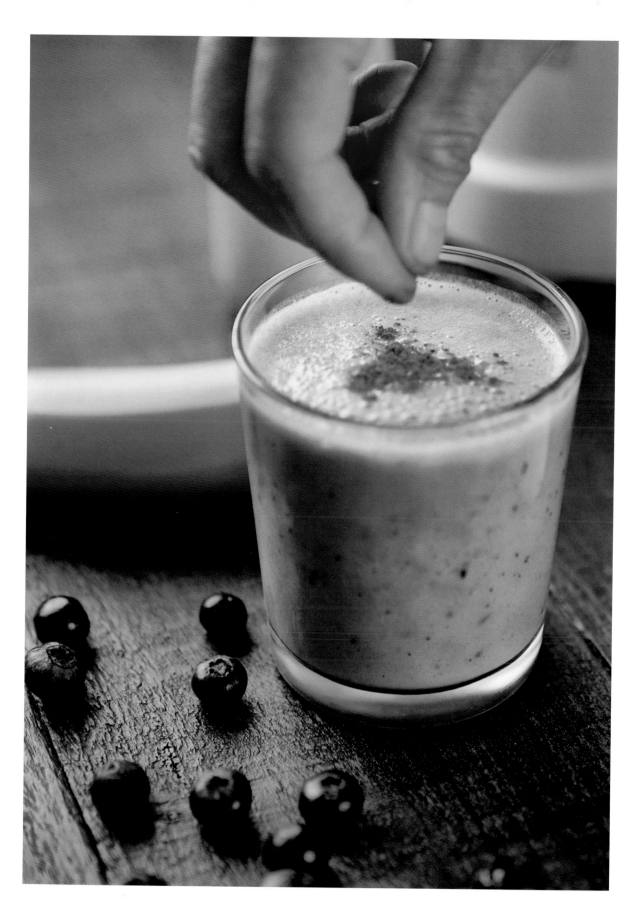

Blueberry 'n' Cinnamon Cream

HOW TO DO IT!

Add the ice to your blender, followed by all other ingredients. Blend for 15 – 30 seconds.

INGREDIENTS:
Serves 1

Ice
1 small handful

Banana
1 small

Blueberries
1 handful

Almond Milk
250 ml

Cinnamon
½ teaspoon

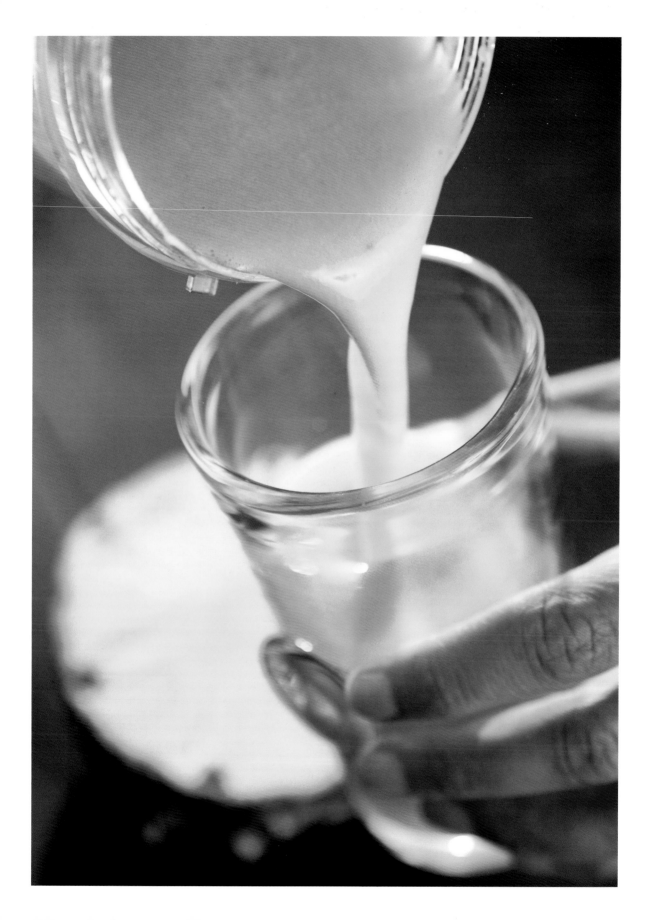

Caribbean Protein
Super Blend

HOW TO DO IT!

Carefully remove the skin and stone from the mango and chop the flesh into small pieces. Peel the pineapple, chop, and discard the hard core. Add the ice to your blender, followed by all other ingredients. Blend for 15 – 30 seconds.

Pea or hemp protein powder are also good alternatives.

INGREDIENTS:
Serves 1

Ice
1 small handful

Mango (ripe)
¼ or 1 small handful

Pineapple
2½ cm slice or 1 handful

Banana
½ small

Coconut Milk (carton)
250 ml

Protein SBM! Powder*
1 tablespoon

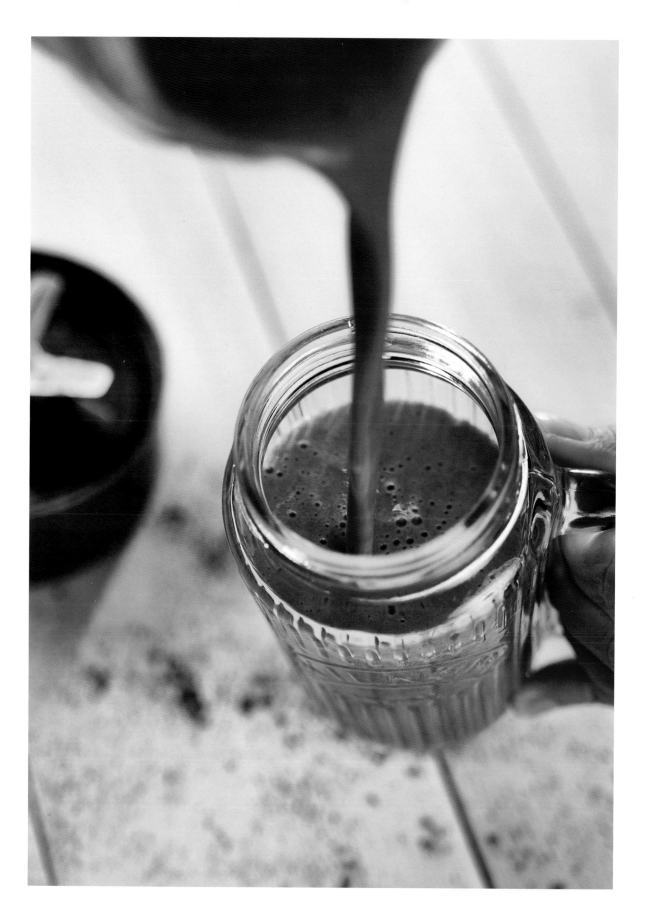

Chocca Mocha Chino

HOW TO DO IT!

Remove the stone from the date. Add the ice to your blender, followed by all other ingredients. Blend for 15 – 30 seconds.

INGREDIENTS:
Serves 1

Ice
1 small handful

Medjool Dates
1

Banana
1 small

Almond Milk
250 ml

Fair Trade Cocoa
1 level teaspoon

Fair Trade Instant Coffee
1 level teaspoon

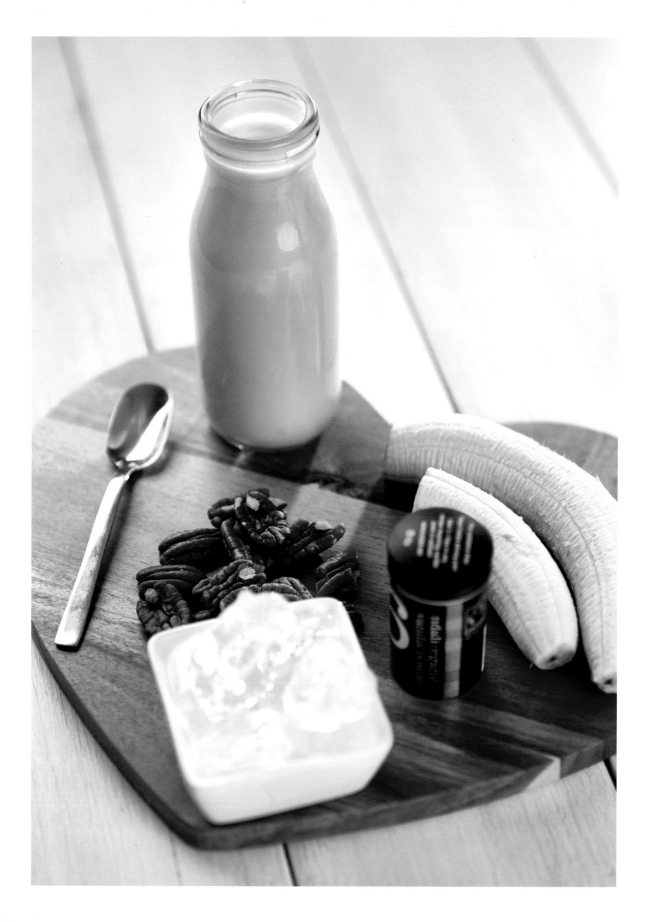

Vanilla Iced Banana Bliss

HOW TO DO IT!

Add the ice to your blender, followed by all other ingredients. Blend for 15 – 30 seconds.

*You could also use vanilla powder or the beans of 1 vanilla pod.

INGREDIENTS:
Serves 1

Ice
1 small handful

Banana
1 ½ small

Pecans
25g or 1 handful

Almond Milk
250 ml

Vanilla Extract*
½ teaspoon

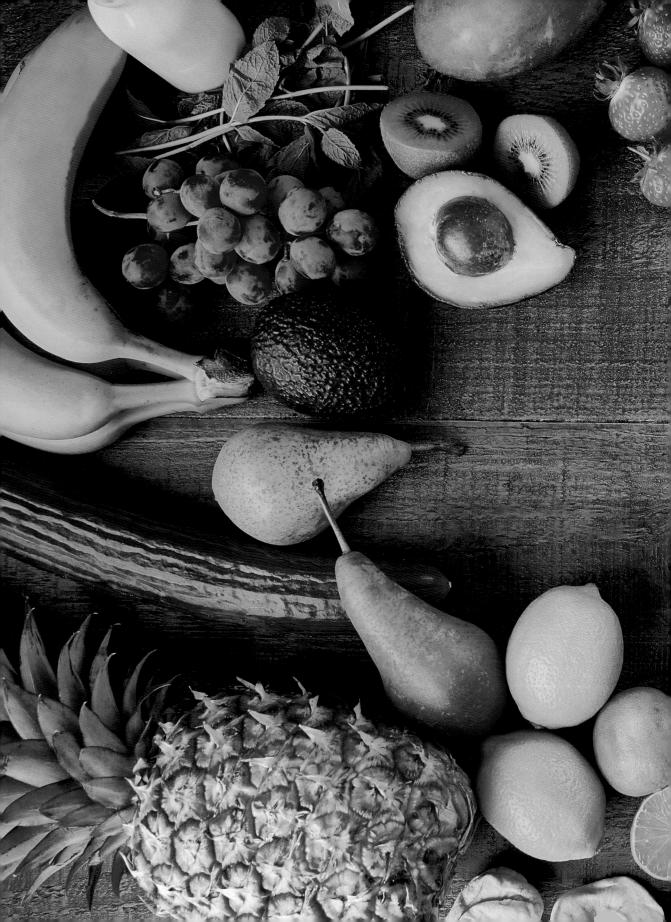

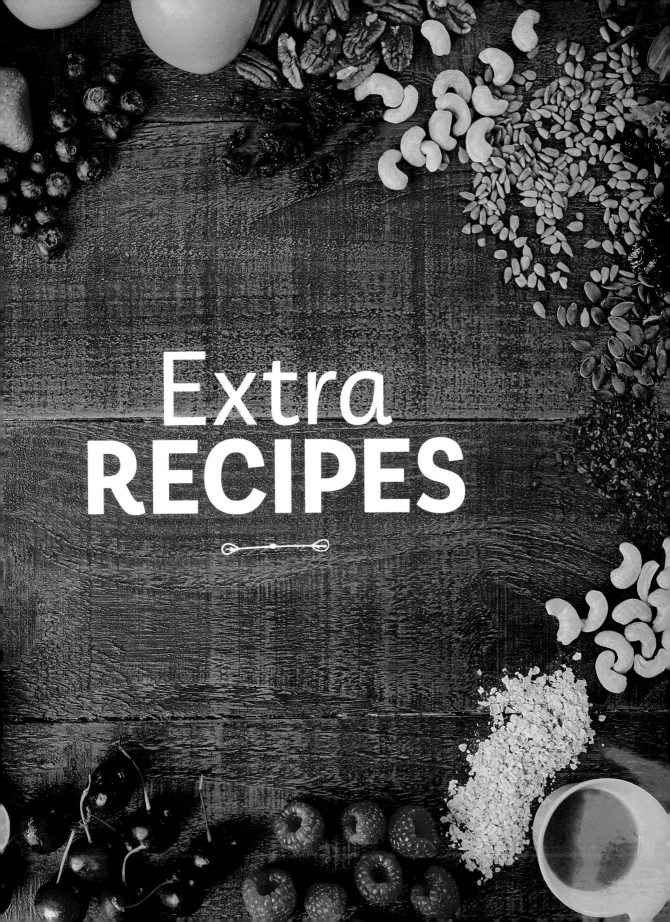

Extra
RECIPES

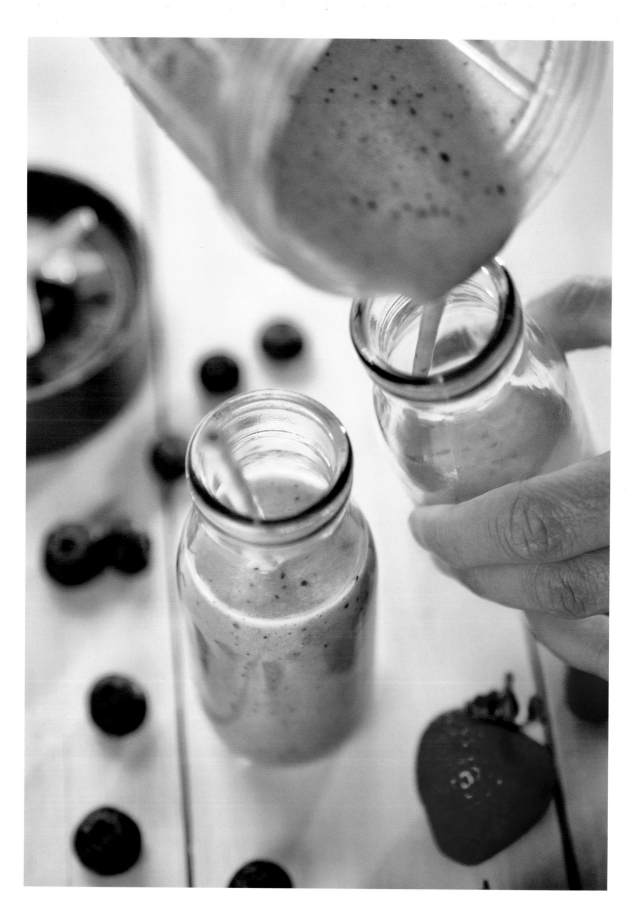

Antioxidant
Super Blend

HOW TO DO IT!

Add the ice to your blender, followed by all other ingredients. Blend for 15 – 30 seconds.

INGREDIENTS:
Serves 1

Ice
1 small handful

Mixed Berries
1 handful

Banana
1 small

Almond Milk
250 ml

Tahini Paste
1 tablespoon

Berry SBM! Powder (optional)
1 teaspoon

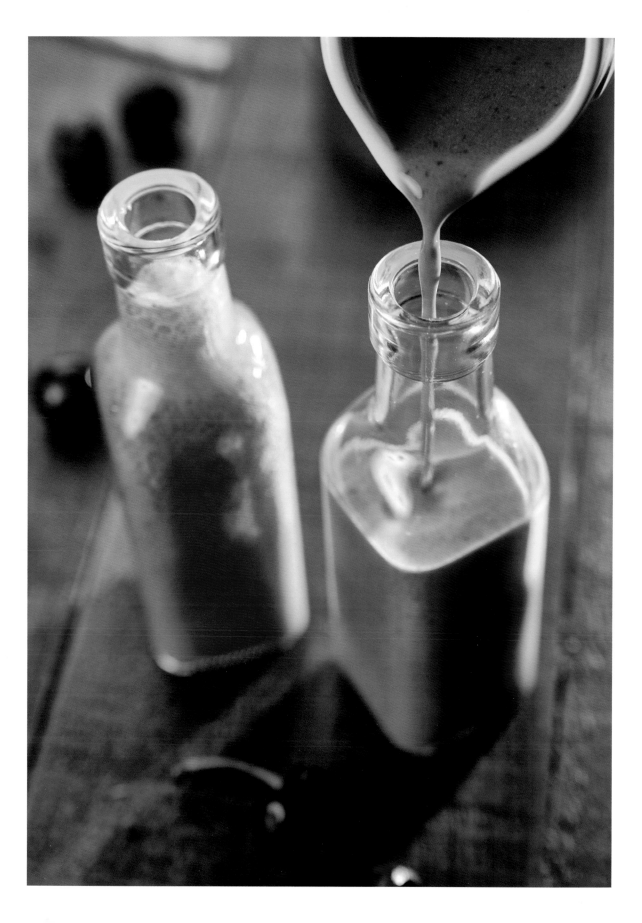

Cherry Vanilla Indulgence

HOW TO DO IT!

Remove the stones from the cherries. Add the ice to your blender, followed by all other ingredients. Blend for 15 – 30 seconds.

*Bio-live, coconut or other alternative.
**You could also use vanilla powder or the beans of 1 vanilla pod.

INGREDIENTS:
Serves 1

Ice
1 small handful

Cherries
12

Yoghurt*
2 tablespoons

Coconut Milk (carton)
300ml

Vanilla Extract**
½ teaspoon

Cashew Butter
1 teaspoon

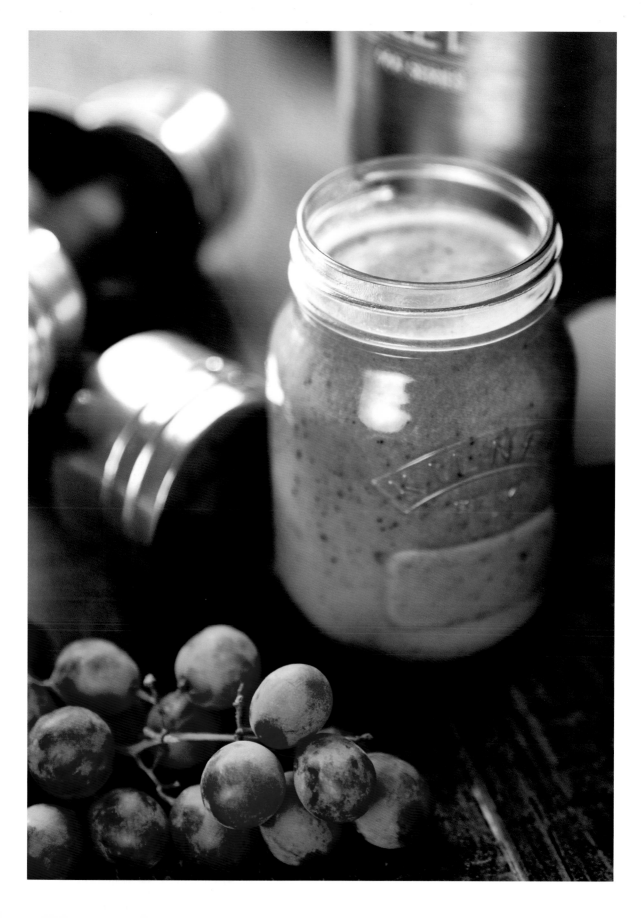

Grape 'n' Blueberry Protein
Super Blend

HOW TO DO IT!

Add the ice to your blender, followed by all other ingredients. Blend for 15 – 30 seconds.

*Bio-live, coconut or other alternative.
**Pea or hemp protein powder are also good alternatives.

INGREDIENTS:
Serves 1

Ice
1 small handful

Red Grapes
1 handful

Blueberries
1 handful

Spinach
1 small handful

Coconut Milk (carton)
200 ml

Yoghurt*
1 tablespoon

Almond Butter
1 teaspoon

Protein SBM! Powder**
1 tablespoon

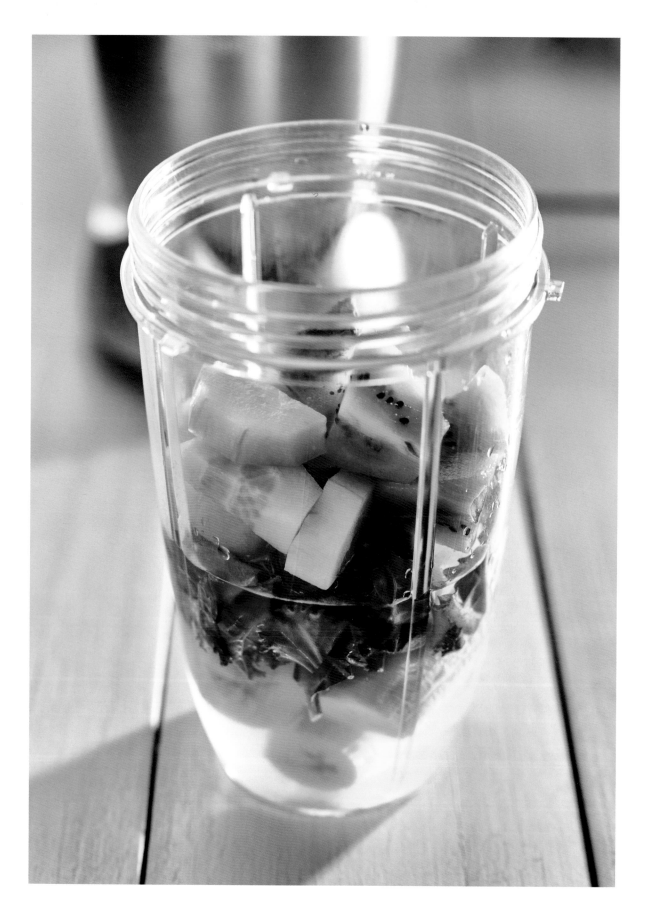

Kiwi, Kale, Cucumber Cooler

HOW TO DO IT!

Remove the skin from the kiwi and cucumber and chop into small chunks. Add the ice to your blender, followed by all the other ingredients. Blend for 15 – 30 seconds.

INGREDIENTS:
Serves 1

Ice
1 small handful

Cucumber
2½ cm chunk or 1 small handful

Kiwi
1

Kale
1 small handful

Banana
1 small

Coconut Water
250 ml

Green SBM! Powder (optional)
1 teaspoon

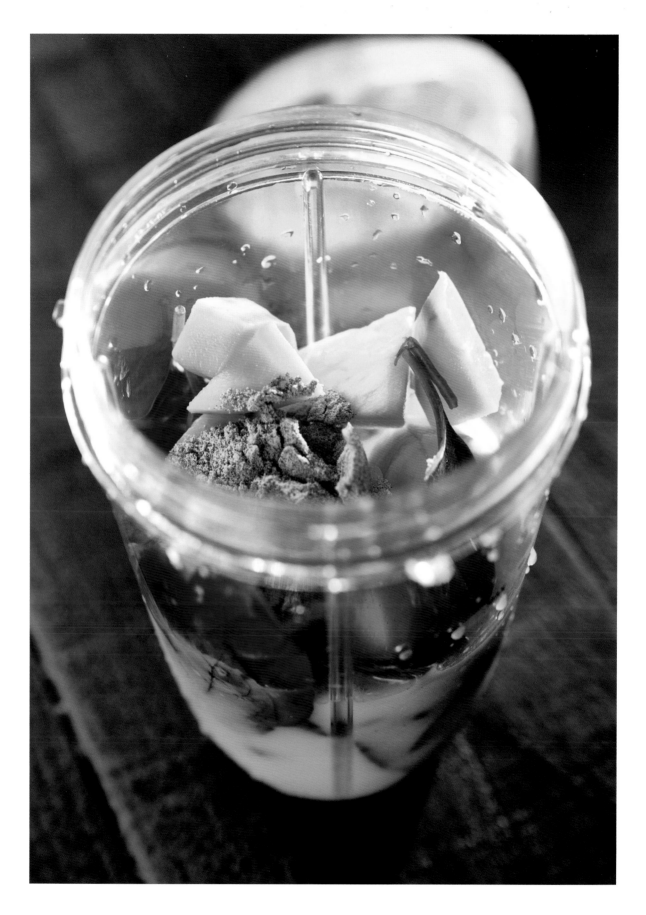

Mango & Banana Protein Super Blend

HOW TO DO IT!

Carefully remove the skin and stone from the mango and chop the flesh into small pieces. Add the ice to your blender, followed by all other ingredients. Blend for 15 – 30 seconds.

*Pea or hemp powder are also good alternatives.

INGREDIENTS:
Serves 1

Ice
1 small handful

Mango (ripe)
¼ or 1 small handful

Banana
1 small

Spinach
1 small handful

Oat Milk
250 ml

Protein SBM! Powder*
1 tablespoon

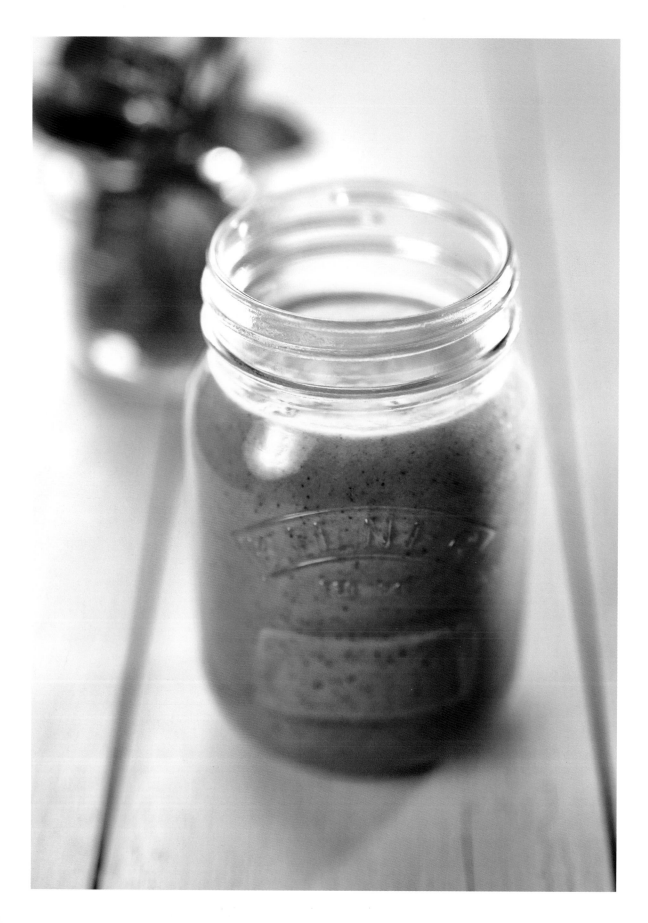

Mighty Minty Mango
Super Blend

HOW TO DO IT!

Carefully remove the skin and stone from the mango and chop the flesh into small pieces. Add the ice to your blender, followed by all other ingredients. Blend for 15 – 30 seconds.

INGREDIENTS:
Serves 1

Ice
1 small handful

Mango (ripe)
½ or 1 large handful

Fresh Mint Leaves
1 large handful

Spinach
1 small handful

Almond Milk
250 ml

Almond Butter
1 teaspoon

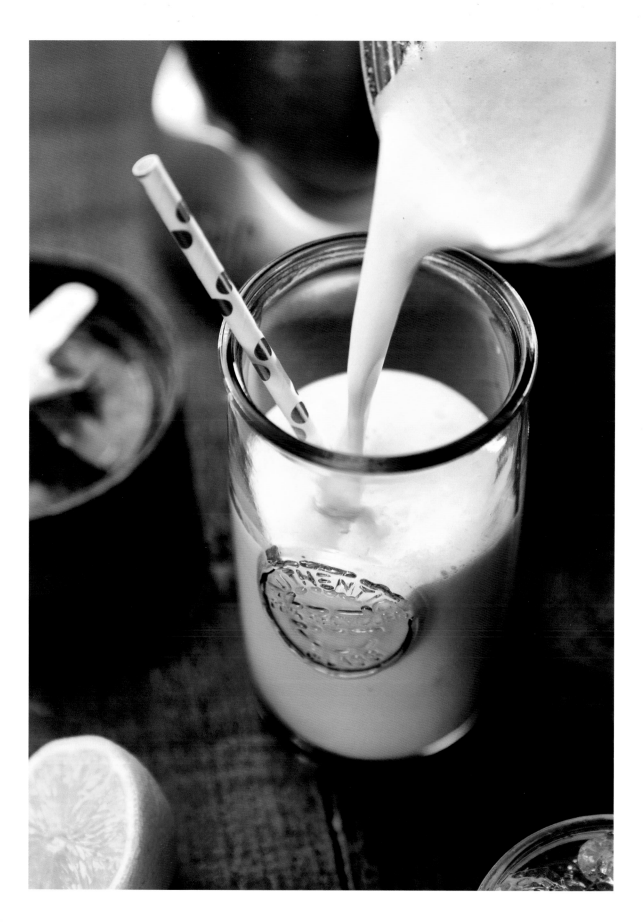

Pineapple Lemon-Aid
Super Blend

HOW TO DO IT!

Peel the pineapple, chop, and discard the hard core. Remove the core from the apple and chop. Remove the skin from the lemon (keep pith on) and chop. Add the ice to your blender, followed by all the other ingredients. Blend for 15 – 30 seconds.

INGREDIENTS:
Serves 1

Ice
1 small handful

Pineapple
2½ cm slice or 1 handful

Apple
½

Lemon
1

Coconut Water
250 ml

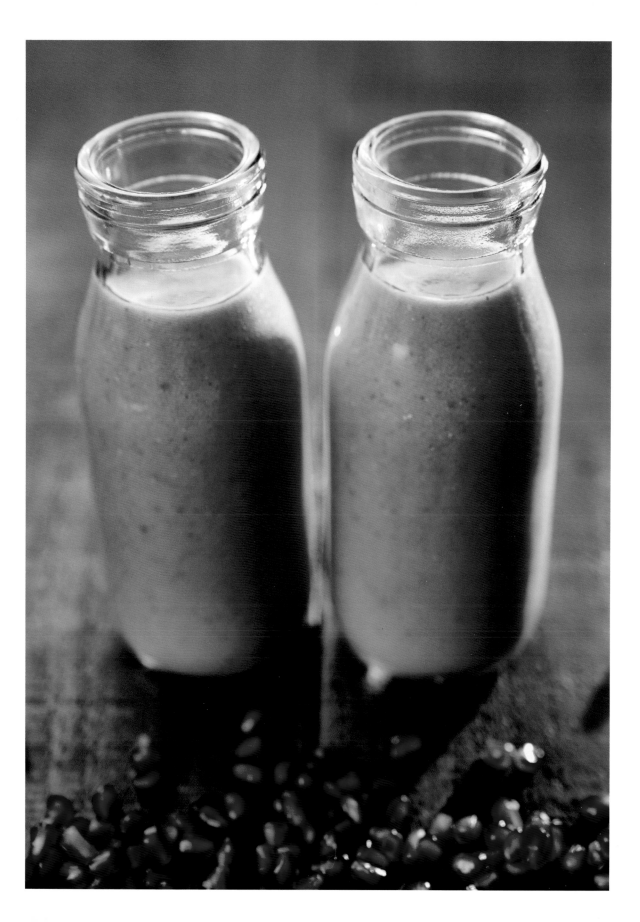

Pom 'n' Pear
Super Shake

HOW TO DO IT!

Remove the core from the pear and chop. Add the ice to your blender, followed by all the other ingredients. Blend for 15 – 30 seconds.

INGREDIENTS:
Serves 1

Ice
1 small handful

Pear
½

Pomegranate Seeds
1 tablespoon

Banana
1 small

Spinach
1 handful

Coconut Milk (carton)
250 ml

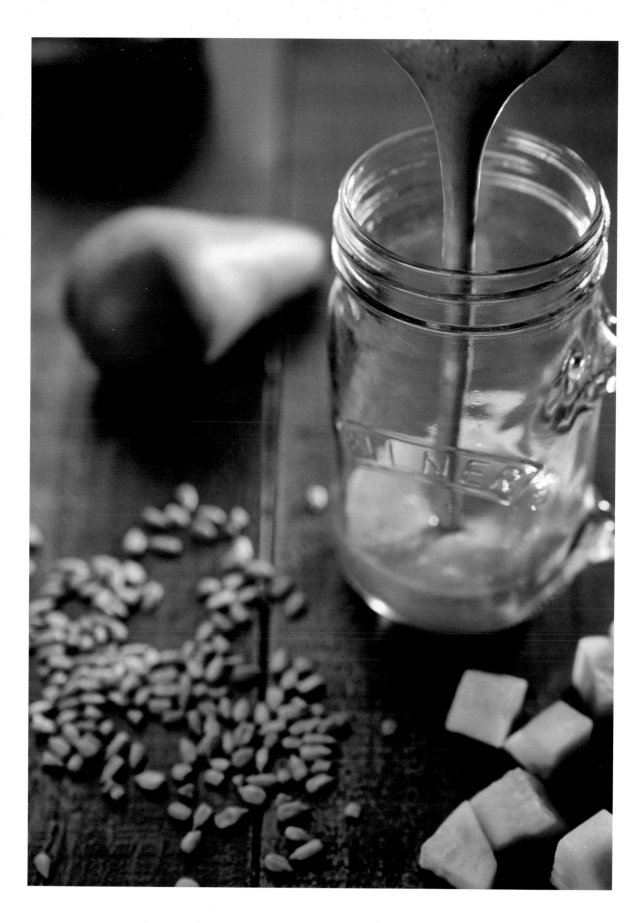

Simple Pear Necessity

HOW TO DO IT!

Remove the core from the pear and chop.
Remove the skin from the cucumber and chop.
Add the ice to your blender, followed by all the
other ingredients. Blend for 15 – 30 seconds.

Bio-live, coconut or other alternative.

INGREDIENTS:
Serves 1

Ice
1 small handful

Pear
1

Cucumber
2½ cm chunk or 1 small handful)

Banana
1 small

Kale
1 small handful

Almond Milk
200 ml

Yoghurt*
1 tablespoon

Sunflower Seeds
1 tablespoon

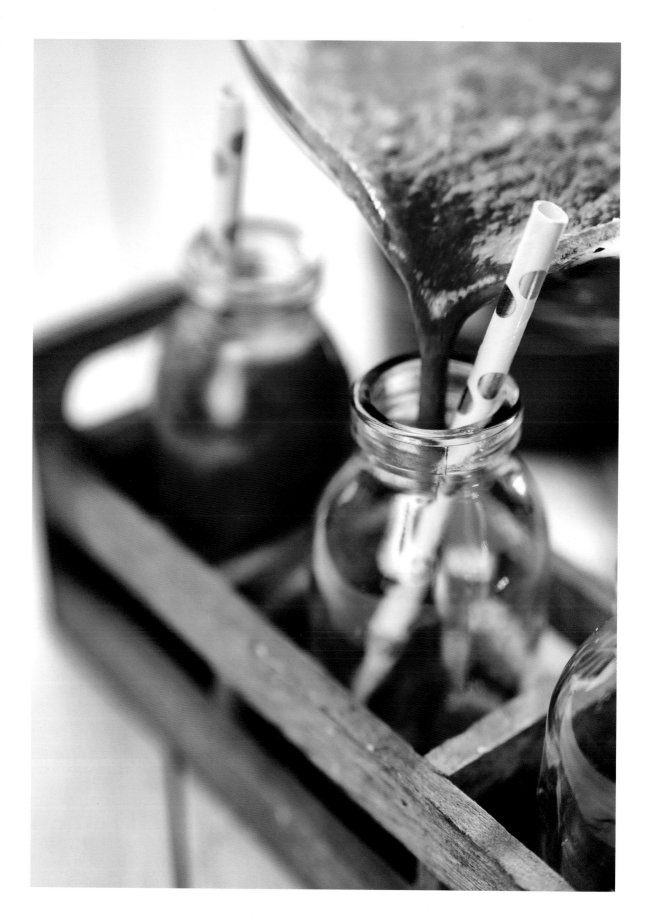

Super Spirulina Smoothie

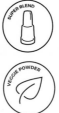

HOW TO DO IT!

Peel the pineapple, chop, and discard the hard core. Add the ice to your blender. Scoop in the flesh of the avocado, followed by all the other ingredients. Blend for 15 – 30 seconds.

INGREDIENTS:
Serves 1

Ice
1 small handful

Pineapple
2½ cm slice or 1 handful

Avocado (ripe)
¼

Kale
1 small handful

Coconut Water
300 ml

Spirulina
1 teaspoon

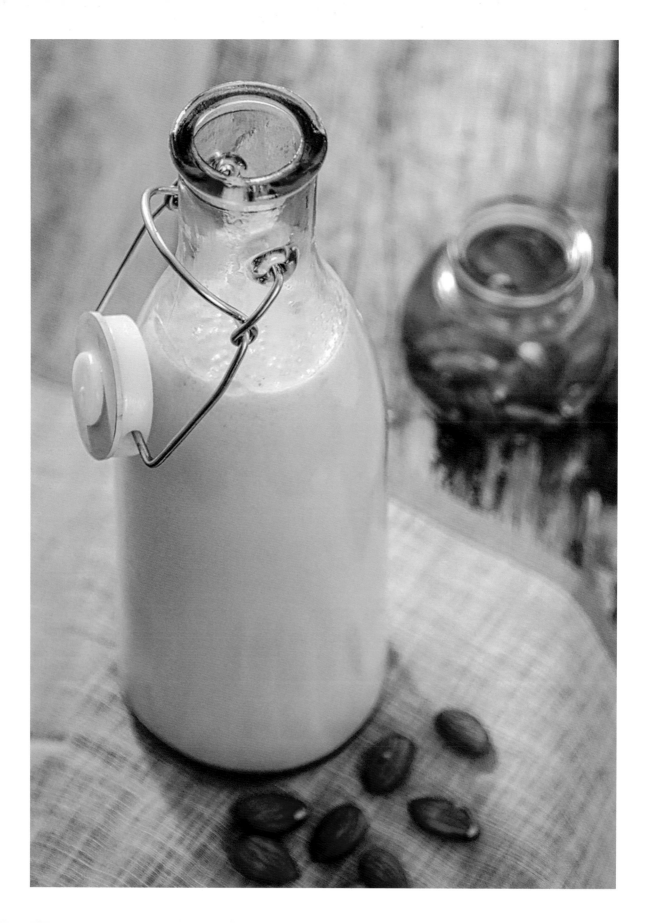

Homemade Milks
(Almond or Oat)

PREPARATION

Soak the almonds in the tap water overnight or for a minimum of 6 hours. Soak the oats in the tap water for about 30 minutes.

HOW TO MAKE

Drain the water and discard. Place the nuts or oats into your blender, pour in the filtered water, salt, and blend for 1 – 2 minutes. Pour the blended milk through either a nut bag or sieve. Discard the pulp and, just like that, you have your milk!
You can also make nut milks using a cold press juicer. For further info check out Jason Vale's **Juice Tube** on YouTube.

INGREDIENTS:
Makes 1 Litre

Almonds or Oats
100 g or 2 handfuls

Tap Water
200 ml

Filtered Water
800 ml

Himalayan Rock Salt
1 pinch

STORAGE

Store in a sealed container in the fridge. **Use within 3 days**. The milk will separate slightly, so just give it a little stir before use.

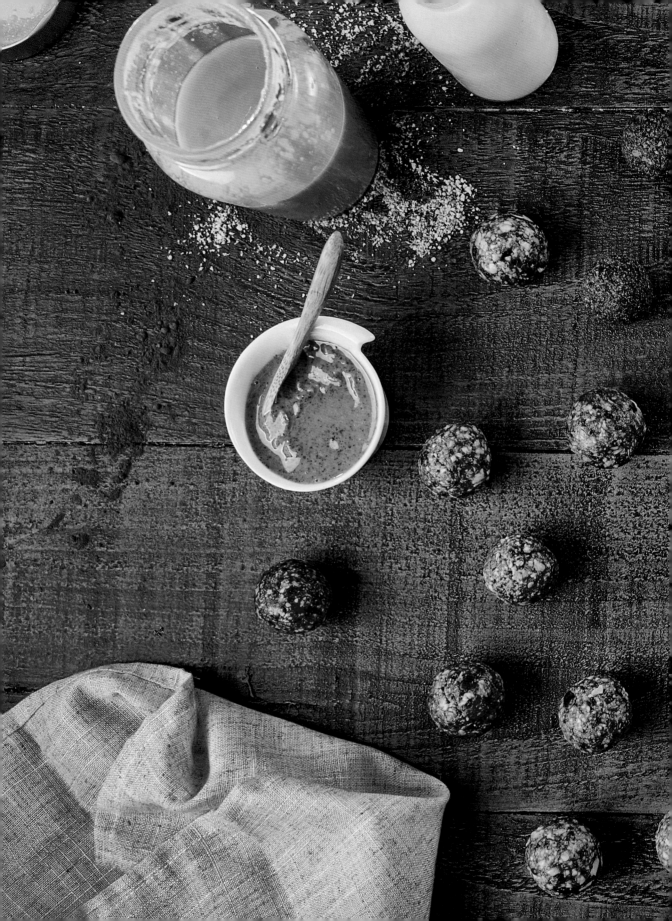

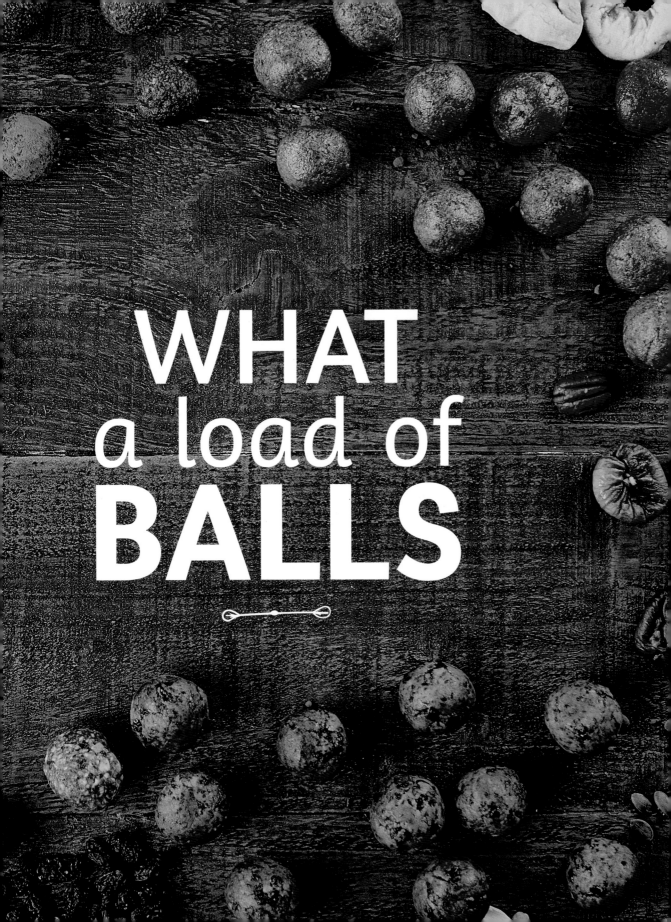

WHAT
a load of
BALLS

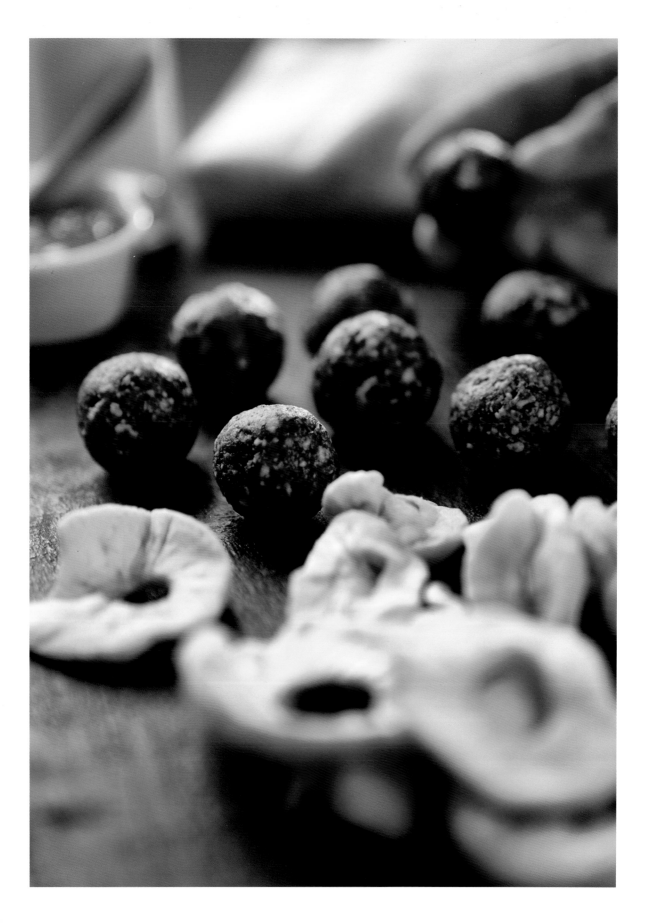

Apple 'n' Pumpkin Seed Power Balls

HOW TO DO IT!

Place all ingredients into the container of a small hand blender and blend for 20 – 30 seconds until combined.

Take a generous teaspoon of mixture and roll into a ball using the palms of your (clean!) hands. Repeat until all the mixture has been used. Pop the balls onto a plate and leave in the fridge for 30 minutes to firm up.

INGREDIENTS:

Serves 8-10

Dried Apple
40 g

Pumpkin Seeds
40 g

Raisins
20 g

Cashew Butter
2 tablespoons

Almond Milk
2 tablespoons

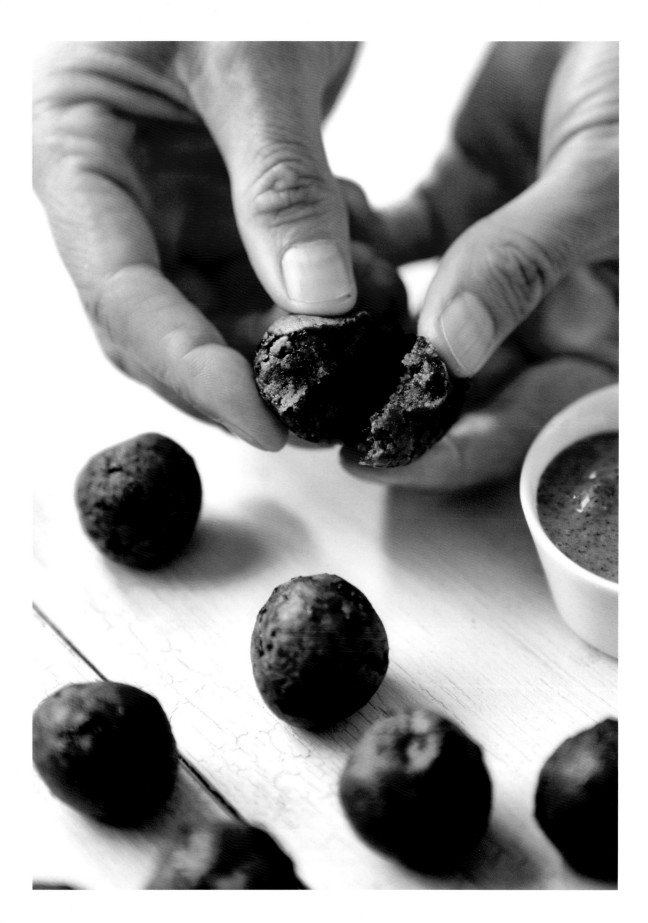

Chewy, Cherry Almond Balls

HOW TO DO IT!

Place all ingredients into the container of a small hand blender and blend for 20 – 30 seconds until combined.

Take a generous teaspoon of mixture and roll into a ball using the palms of your (clean!) hands. Repeat until all the mixture has been used. Pop the balls onto a plate and leave in the fridge for 30 minutes to firm up.

INGREDIENTS:
Serves 8-10

Ground Almonds
60 g

Dried Cherries
60 g

Almond Butter
1 tablespoon

Almond Milk
2 tablespoons

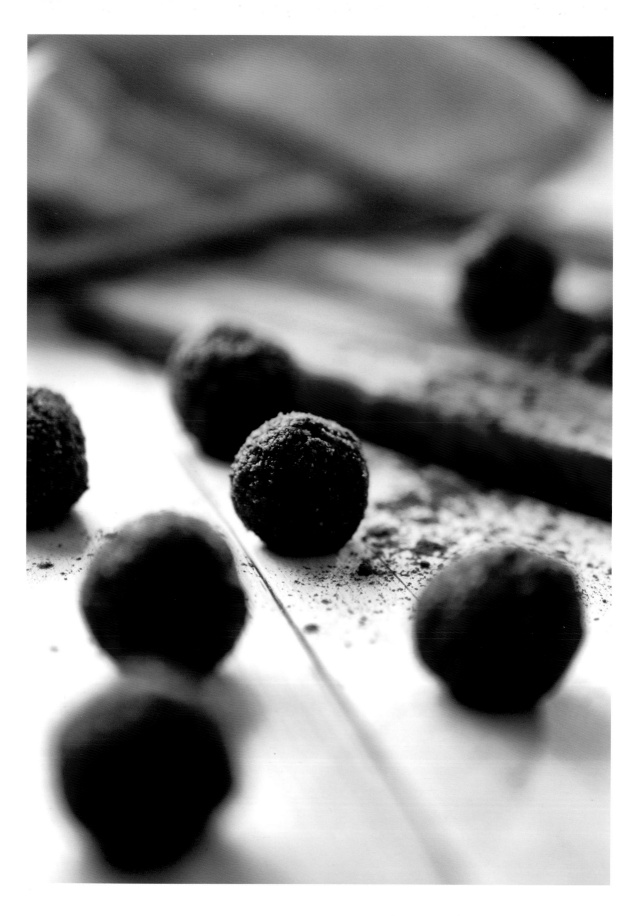

Chilli Cocoa Power Balls

HOW TO DO IT!

Remove the stones from the dates. Place the cashews into the container of a small hand blender and blitz for 10 – 20 seconds. Add in all other ingredients and blend for 20 – 30 seconds until combined.

Take a generous teaspoon of mixture and roll into a ball using the palms of your (clean!) hands. Repeat until all the mixture has been used. Pop the balls onto a plate and leave in the fridge for 30 minutes to firm up.

INGREDIENTS:
Serves 8-10

Medjool Dates
2

Cashew nuts
70 g

Raisins
20 g

Fair Trade Cocoa
1 heaped teaspoon

Chilli
1 pinch

Almond Milk
2 tablespoons

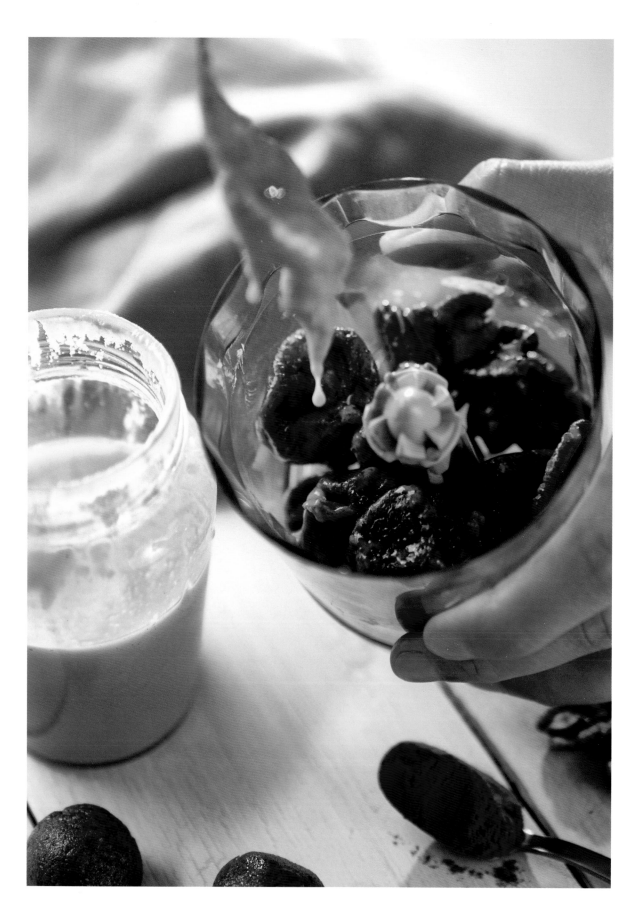

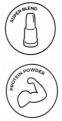

Pecan
Power Balls

HOW TO DO IT!

Place the pecans into the container of a small hand blender and blitz for 10 – 20 seconds. Remove the hard ends from the figs. Add in all other ingredients and blend for 20 – 30 seconds until combined.

Take a generous teaspoon of mixture and roll into a ball using the palms of your (clean!) hands. Repeat until all the mixture has been used. Pop the balls onto a plate and leave in the fridge for 30 minutes to firm up.

Pea or hemp protein powder are also good alternatives.

INGREDIENTS:
Serves 8-10

Pecan Nuts
60 g

Dried Figs
50 g

Tahini Paste
1 tablespoon

Cashew Butter
1 tablespoon

Cinnamon
1 teaspoon

Protein SBM! Powder*
1 tablespoon

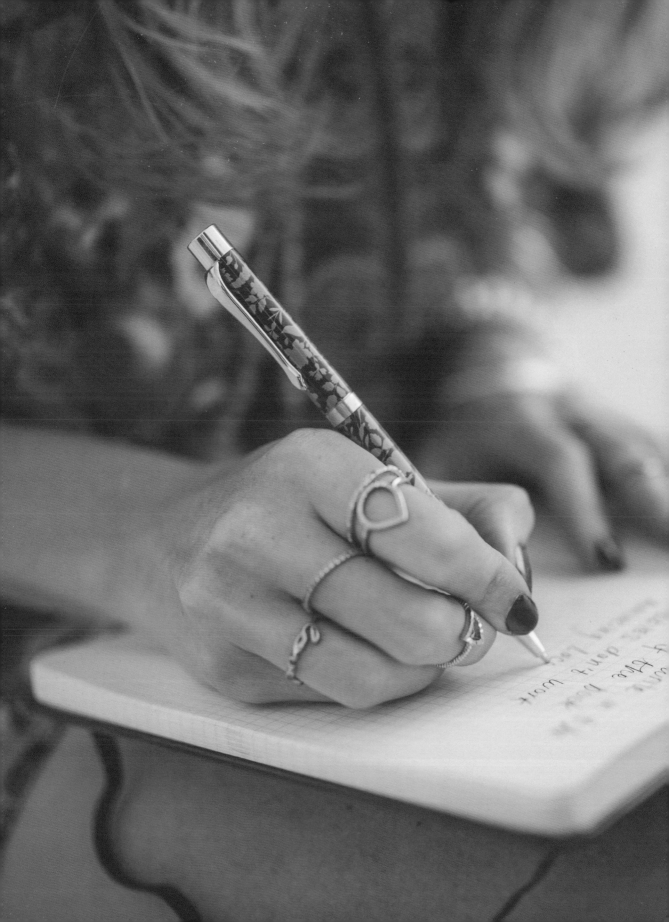

My
SUPER
BLEND
ME!
Journal

IF YOUR LIFE'S WORTH LIVING,
IT'S WORTH RECORDING

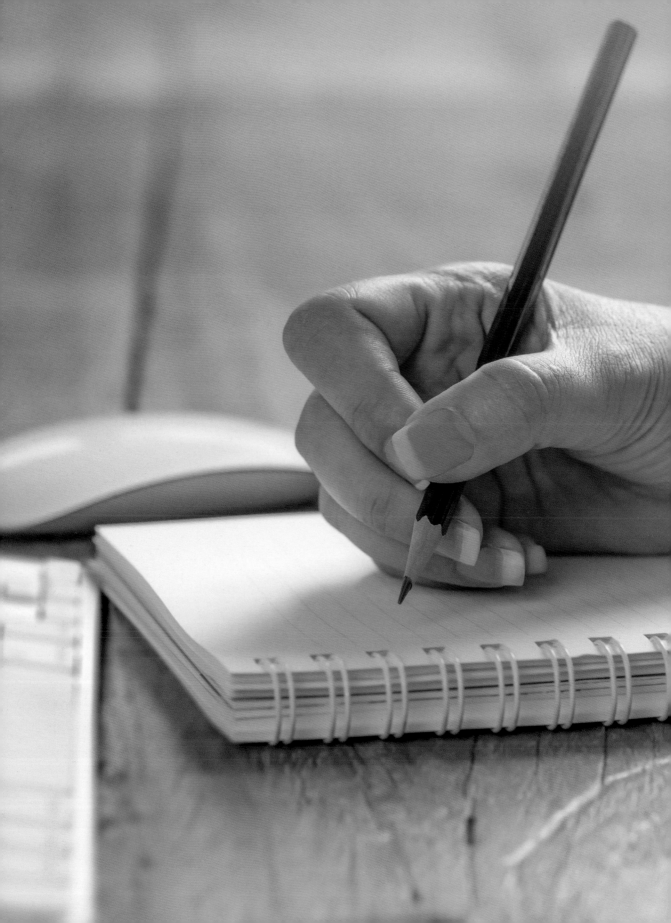

I have found over the years that if you keep a journal of some kind whilst doing a challenge of this nature, you are more engaged with it.

H aving said that, I am aware this process won't be for everyone. What I would say is that even if you don't fancy filling in (or filling out, if you're from the US!) your journal, please make a point of recording your *before* and *after* stats. You will be *genuinely* amazed at the magnitude of difference in such a short space of time, not only in weight (if you are doing this for weight loss) but in how you feel and overall body stats. Muscle is heavier than fat but takes up far less room, so some people see little change on the scales but a huge change on the 'inches lost' front and overall body shape. If you get a chance, please share your results with us at *results@superblendme. com* as by taking a small amount of time to record a short video, or send in your photos and stats, you could potentially inspire many people from all over the world to change their lives. If you manage to do this, I'd like to personally thank you in advance; you're helping to make a huge difference.

If you are the kind of person who loves the idea of fully engaging with the experience, then keeping a journal is the perfect way to do this, which is why I have laid out a full 21-day *Super Blend Me!* journal. Clearly, if you are doing a shorter challenge, as most will be, then just fill in the days you are doing.

DOWNLOAD YOUR JOURNAL

If you have the e-book version and your device won't allow you to write within the e-book, then don't worry as you can download a free PDF version at *www. superblendme.com*

GET A SHARPIE!

My final piece of 'journal related' advice is to get a Sharpie, or any other pen which will allow you to write on the glossy pages with ease.

GOOD LUCK!

BEFORE

HEIGHT	
WEIGHT	
BODY SHAPE	
BODY FAT %	
MUSCLE %	
WAIST MEASUREMENT	
CHEST MEASUREMENT	
HIP MEASUREMENT	
AVERAGE EXCERCISE PER WEEK	
TYPE OF EXERCISE	

BRIEFLY DESCRIBE YOUR HEALTH AND HOW YOU FEEL BEFORE STARTING...

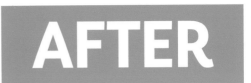

HEIGHT	
WEIGHT	
BODY SHAPE	
BODY FAT %	
MUSCLE %	
WAIST MEASUREMENT	
CHEST MEASUREMENT	
HIP MEASUREMENT	
AVERAGE EXCERCISE PER WEEK	
TYPE OF EXERCISE	

FINISH THIS SENTENCE; 'I HAVE COMPLETED THE SUPER BLEND ME! PLAN AND I FEEL...'

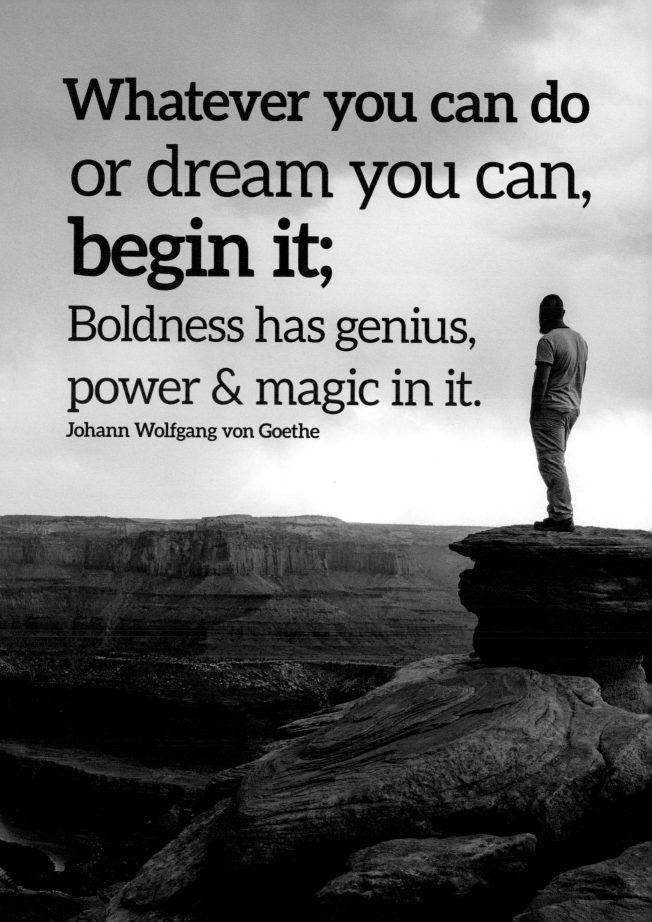

Whatever you can do
or dream you can,
begin it;
Boldness has genius,
power & magic in it.
Johann Wolfgang von Goethe

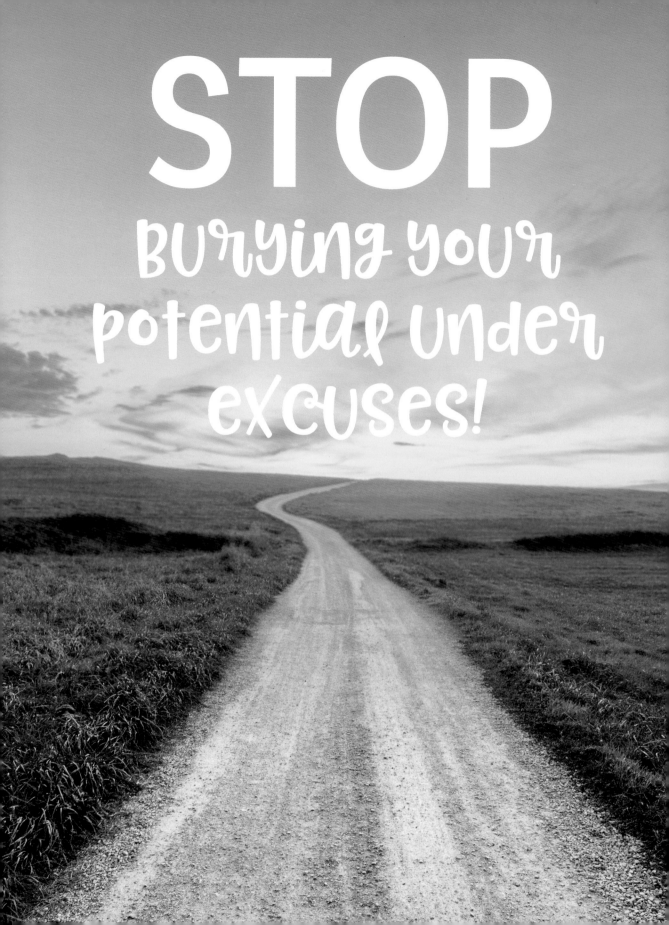

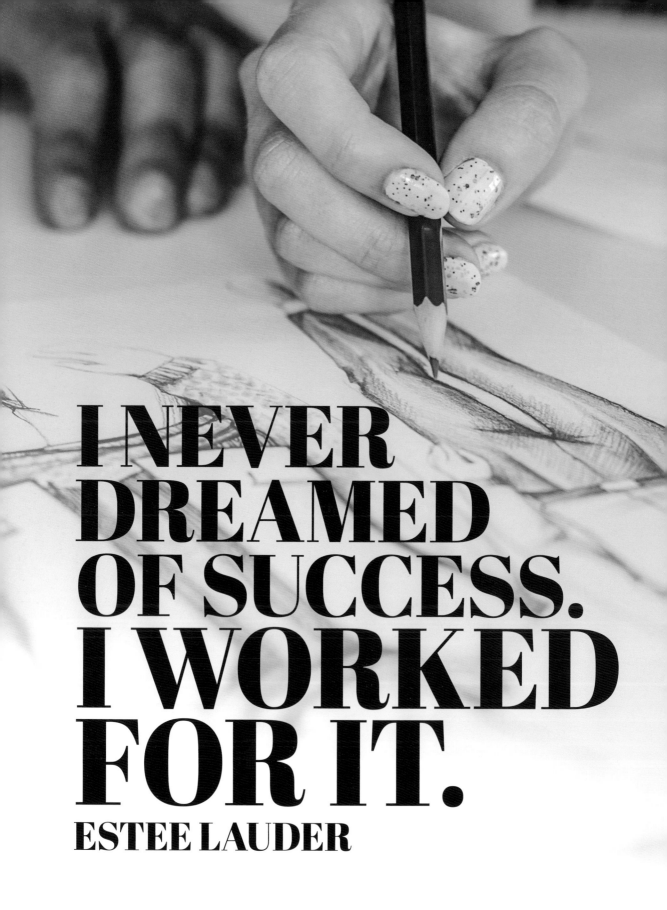

I NEVER DREAMED OF SUCCESS. I WORKED FOR IT.

ESTEE LAUDER

DAY 3

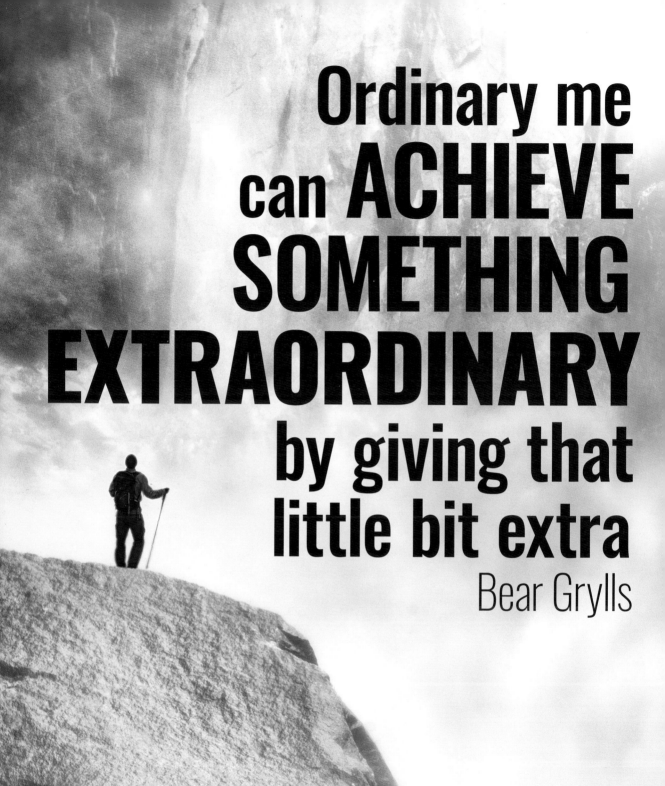

Ordinary me can **ACHIEVE SOMETHING EXTRAORDINARY** by giving that little bit extra

Bear Grylls

DAY 4

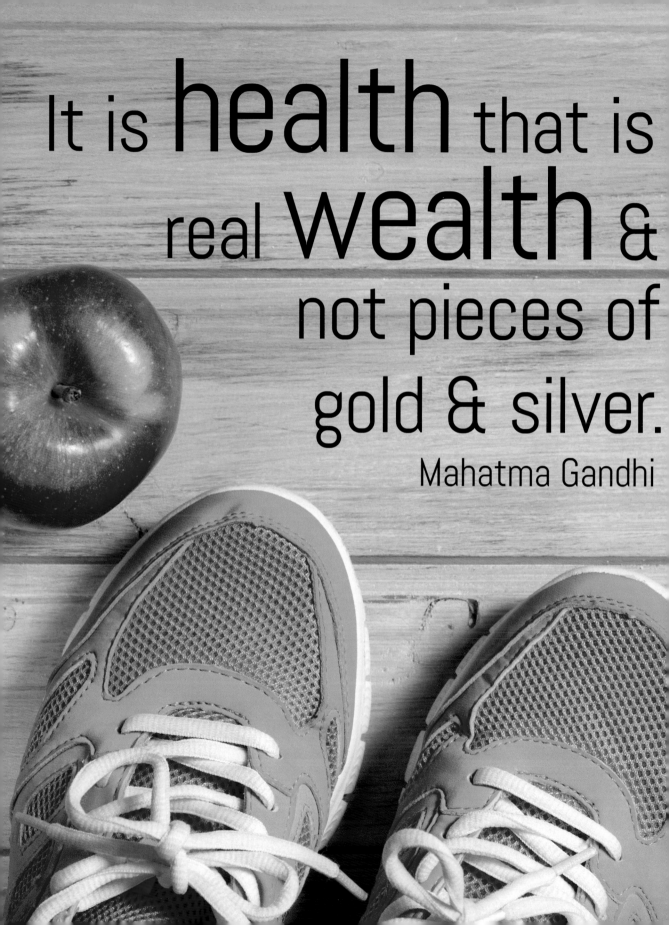

It is health that is real wealth & not pieces of gold & silver.
Mahatma Gandhi

DAY 5

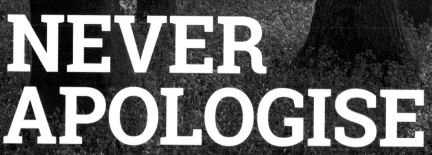

NEVER APOLOGISE

for having high standards.
People who really want to be in your life

WILL RISE UP TO MEET THEM.

You either get bitter or you get better. It's that simple. You either take what has been dealt to you and allow it to make you a better person, or you allow it to tear you down. The choice does not belong to fate, it belongs to you.

CONGRATULATIONS
IT'S DAY 7!

If you set yourself the goal of completing the 7-day *Super Blend Me! Challenge* then congratulations are in order – it's your last day! Please remember to read the *Life After Super Blend Me!* section (page 219) so you're fully prepared for the next stage, and to ensure all of your hard work doesn't go to waste the second your challenge comes to an end. Tomorrow is Results Day so don't forget to record your stats (page 175) and / or email them to *results@superblendme.com*. You may, of course, be feeling so good and so in the *Super Blend Me!* zone that although you originally set out to do just 7 days, you're now tempted to do a little cheeky extension to make it a 10-day challenge or even longer. Whatever you decide, congratulations on doing whatever it took to reach your 7-day goal. If all has gone according to plan, you should be feeling and looking a whole lot better than you did at the start.

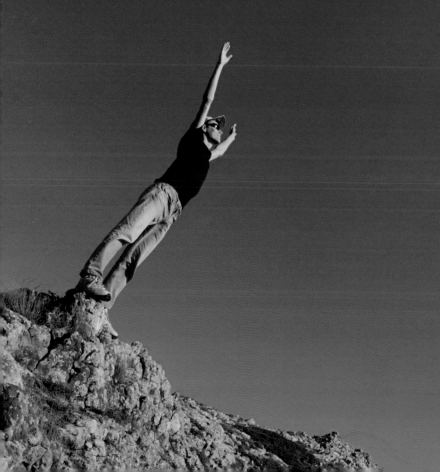

"OBSTACLES ARE DESIGNED TO MAKE YOU **STRONGER**, ONLY THE WEAK AVOID THEM."

DAY 8

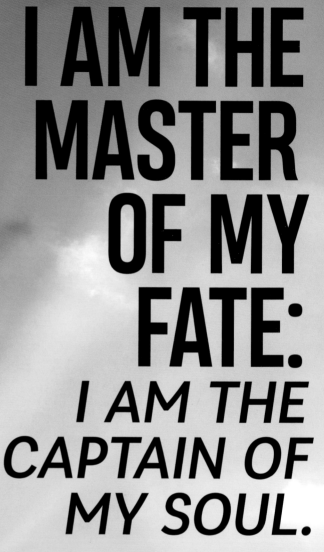

I AM THE MASTER OF MY FATE:

I AM THE CAPTAIN OF MY SOUL.

William Ernest Henley

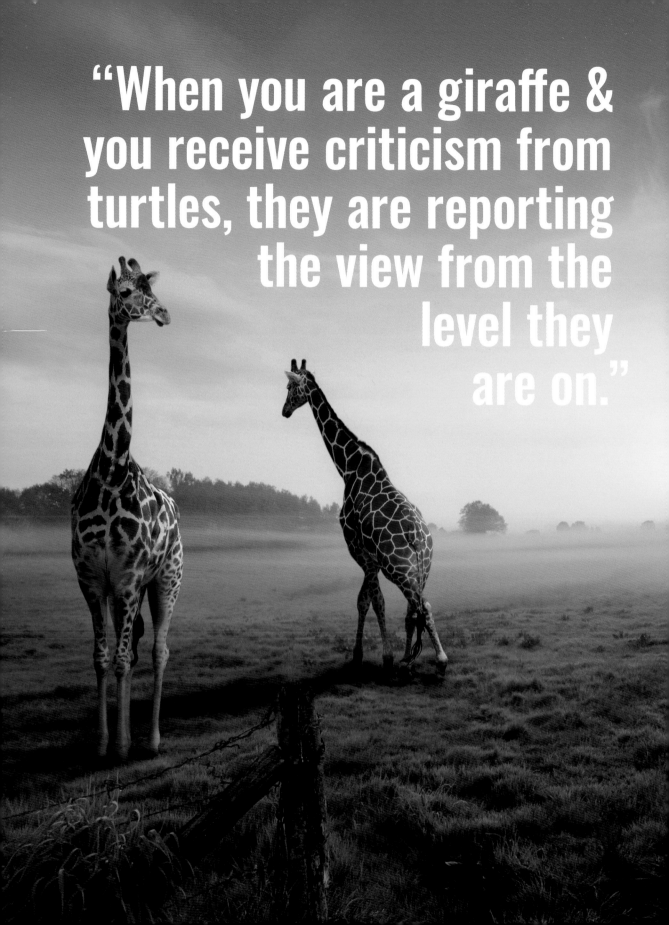

"When you are a giraffe & you receive criticism from turtles, they are reporting the view from the level they are on."

CONGRATULATIONS
IT'S DAY 10!

If you set yourself the goal of completing the 10-day *Super Blend Me! Challenge* then huge congratulations are in order – it's your final day on nothing but *Super Blends*. Please remember to read the *Life After Super Blend Me!* section (page 219) so you're fully prepared for the next stage, and to ensure all of your hard work doesn't go to waste the second your challenge comes to an end. Tomorrow is Results Day so don't forget to record your stats (page 175) and / or email them to *results@superblendme. com.* I personally love reading the results, especially as it's not just about weight loss, so think about your overall health and how this may have changed. Your results also help to inspire others from all over the world. If you don't get a chance to email them in, then you can always jump on my social media channels and post there. Congratulations for setting a goal and doing whatever it took to make sure you completed it.

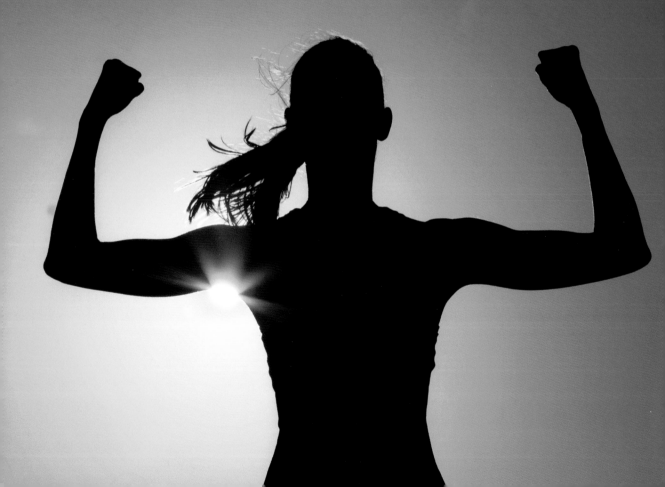

Be **STRONG** when you are weak, **BRAVE** when you are scared, and **HUMBLE** when you are victorious.

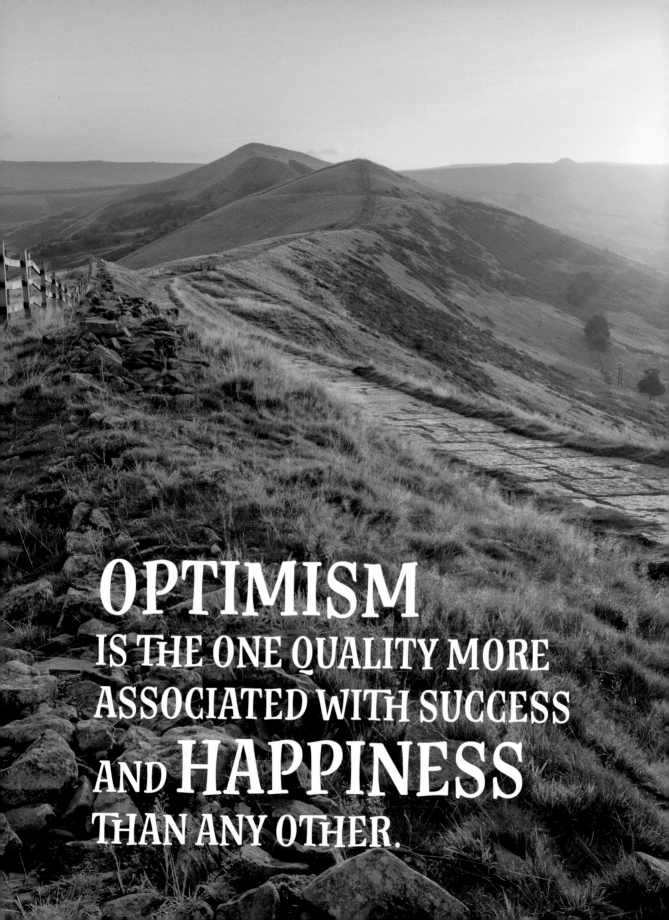

OPTIMISM
IS THE ONE QUALITY MORE
ASSOCIATED WITH SUCCESS
AND **HAPPINESS**
THAN ANY OTHER.

DAY 12

What you get by **achieving your goals** is not as important as what **you become** by achieving your goals.

Henry David Thoreau

DAY 13

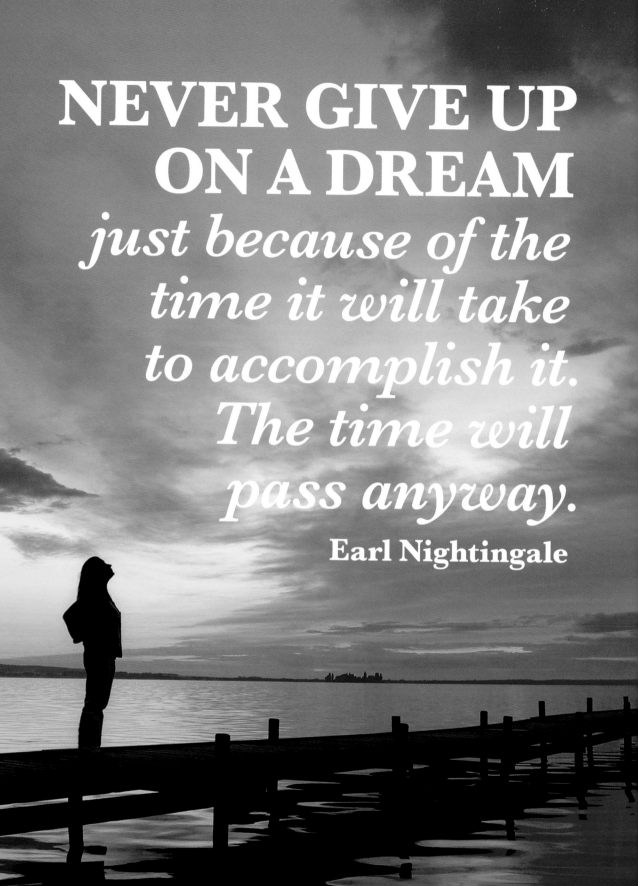

CONGRATULATIONS
IT'S DAY 14!

If you set yourself the goal of completing the 14-day *Super Blend Me! Challenge* then huge congratulations are in order - it's your final day on nothing but Super Blends. Please remember to read the *Life After Super Blend Me!* section (page 219) so you're fully prepared for the next stage, and to ensure all of your hard work doesn't go to waste the second your challenge comes to an end. Tomorrow is Results Day so don't forget to record your stats (page 175) and / or email them to *results@superblendme. com*. I personally love reading the results, especially as it's not just about weight loss, so think about your overall health and how this may have changed. Your results also help to inspire others from all over the world. If you don't get a chance to email them in, then you can always jump on my social media channels and post there. Congratulations for setting a goal and doing whatever it took to make sure you completed it. People get great results on a 7-day *Super Blend Me! Challenge*, but when you raise the game to 14 days like you have – you should be seeing some pretty significant changes!

DO IT WITH PASSION OR NOT AT ALL

Either I WILL FIND A WAY or CREATE A WAY; **BUT I WILL NOT CREATE AN EXCUSE**

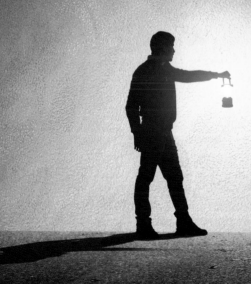

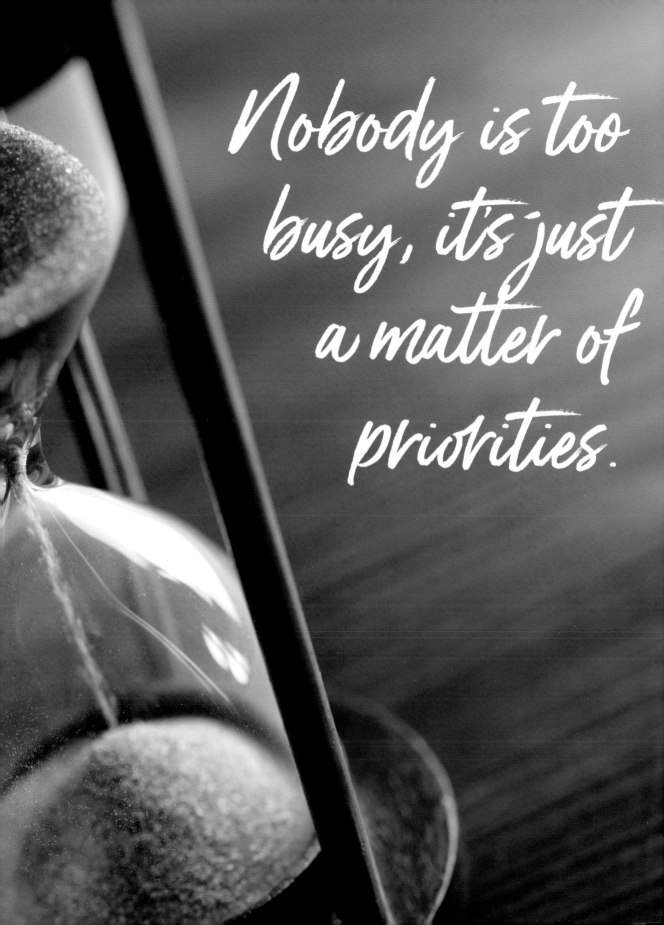

Nobody is too busy, it's just a matter of priorities.

TAKE CARE OF YOUR BODY. IT'S THE ONLY PLACE YOU HAVE TO LIVE.

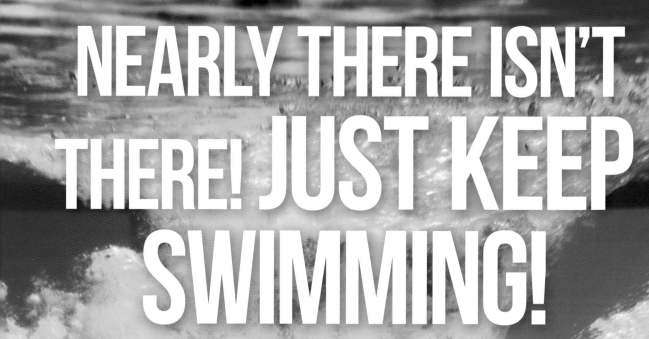
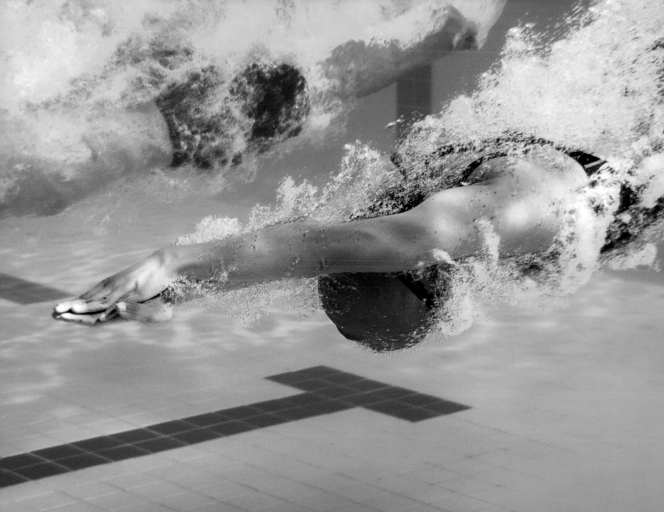

NEARLY THERE ISN'T THERE! JUST KEEP SWIMMING!

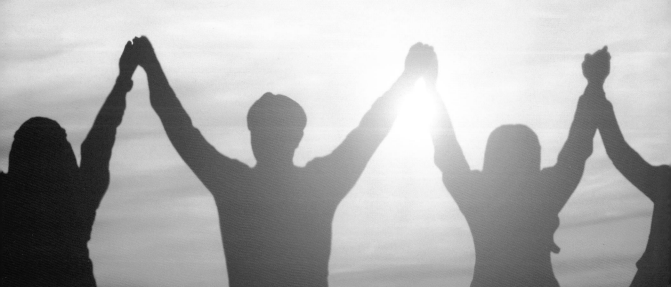

Successful people do what they need to do whether they like it or not

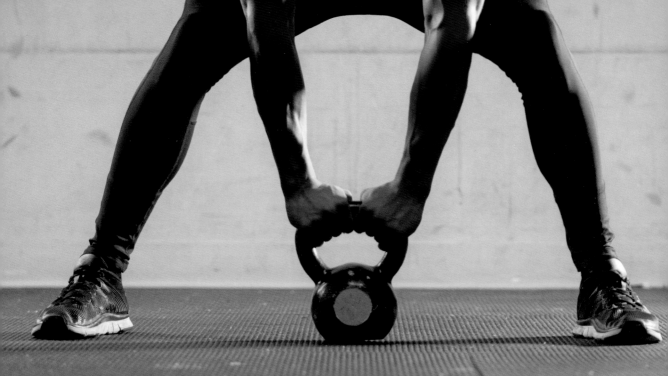

YOU DIDN'T COME THIS FAR TO ONLY COME THIS FAR

CONGRATULATIONS
IT'S DAY 21!

If you set yourself the goal of the big 21-day *Super Blend Me! Challenge* then a MASSIVE congratulations is in order – it's your final day on nothing but *Super Blends* and you're no doubt more than ready to start using your teeth again! To make sure you come off the plan in the right way, please remember to read the *Life After Super Blend Me!* section TODAY (page 219), not only to fully prepare you for the next stage, but also to make sure all of your hard work doesn't go to waste the second your challenge comes to an end. Tomorrow is Results Day so don't forget to record your stats (page 175) and / or email them to *results@superblendme.com*. I personally love reading the results, especially as it's not just about weight loss, so think about your overall health and how this may have changed. Your results also help to inspire others from all over the world. If you don't get a chance to email them in, then you can always jump on my social media channels and post there. Congratulations for setting a goal and doing whatever it took to make sure you completed it. People get great results on a 7-day *Super Blend Me! Challenge*, but when you raise the game to 21 days like you have – you should be seeing some pretty significant changes.

LIFE AFTER
SUPER BLEND ME!

PUTTING YOU IN CHARGE!

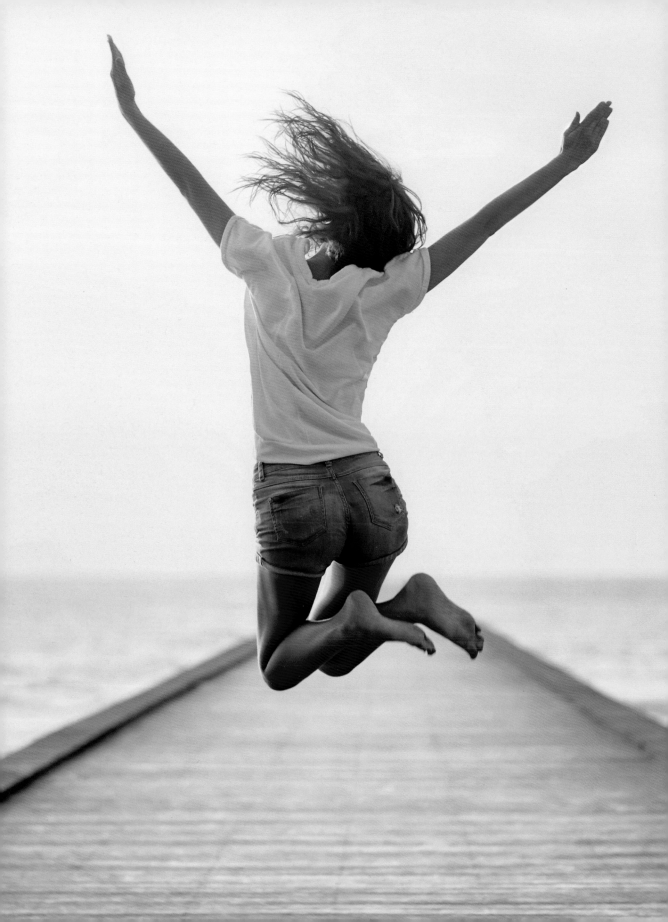

CONGRATULATIONS YOU'VE DONE IT!

...now don't f**k it up!

THE POWER OF POSITIVE MOMENTUM

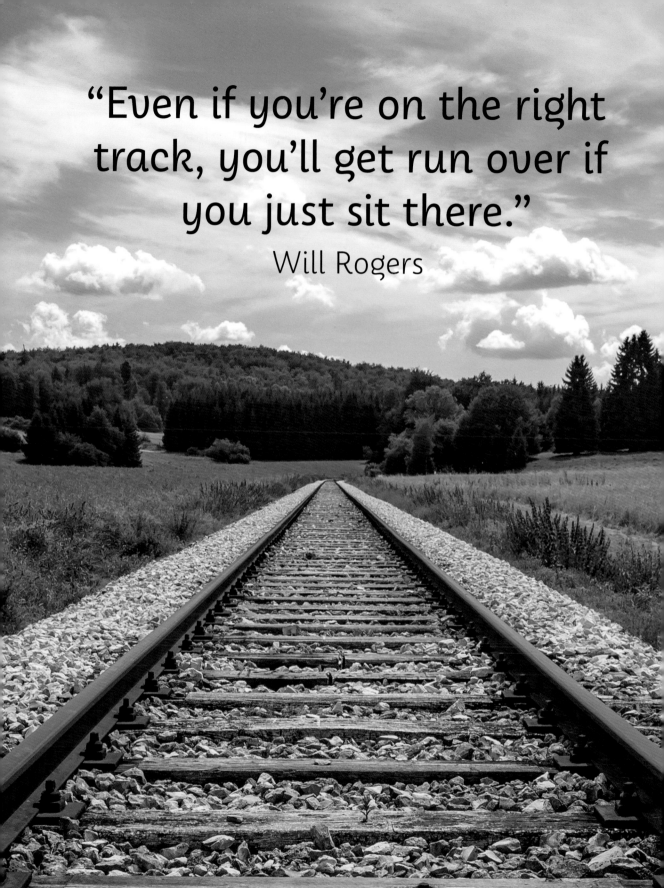

"Even if you're on the right track, you'll get run over if you just sit there."

Will Rogers

Let me be the first to congratulate you on completing your Super Blend Me! Challenge.

I know the reasons for initially taking it on will vary from person to person. Some may have used it as a quick shredding exercise and others to kick-start a major lifestyle change. However, one thing is for sure, if you followed the plan to the letter and abided by the *7 Rules* and *7 Tips For Success*, you will be feeling a little lighter, leaner and sharper than you did before you started. I am also sure that whether you took on the quick 7-day *Super Blend Me! Challenge* or you went for the full-on 21-day *Super Blend Me! Challenge*, the last thing you'll want to happen is for all of your dedication, commitment and focus to go out of the window the second the challenge ends. This is why it is so important to maximise and really harness the positive momentum you have built over the course of the challenge. The good news is you can gain positive momentum in a relatively short space of time (as you will have seen). But you also need to be aware that it can be lost in a heartbeat, too. My advice, while you are feeling good and have this wonderful momentum behind you, is to take *full advantage* of it.

No matter what length of challenge you opted for, or the reasons behind it, how you follow on from your *Super Blend Me! Challenge* is extremely important. You have been on a highly nutritious, liquid-based diet for a significant length of time and what you eat, particularly during the first couple of days, is very important. This is why I have included this after-plan section, plus the 5 *Cheeky Ways To Stay On Track* (page 243) to make sure you're not left high and dry after you finish your challenge. Before we go into the specific after-plan options available to you I wish to give an overview of some of the key nutritional principles, and some advice that you may find useful should you wish to design your own follow-on plan , moving forward. To that end, my first major piece of advice is...

DON'T EAT A FAMILY SIZE KFC BUCKET AS YOUR FIRST MEAL!

Now, I am sure this is the last thing you'd ever do, but I need to cover it as this is precisely what someone did after they spent two weeks filming a show called *Celebrity Detox*.

The show aired in the UK back in 2003, and just when you thought reality TV had gone just about as low as it could go, this little gem came along. The show followed a bunch of celebrities as they spent two weeks on a very strict detox, which even included them giving themselves enemas (which they filmed!). It was reported that one of the celebs had had such a craving for KFC (the entire time) that the first thing he did when he got to the airport on the way home was order, and eat, an entire family sized Kentucky Fried Chicken bucket.

The problem was, his body was now so clean and his stomach simply not used to that amount of excess food going in, that he suffered...a lot! He ended up in excruciating pain and was 'stuck' (if you know what I mean) for a long time. Once you have followed a detox your body becomes far more sensitive to what it deems as *foreign invaders* and will immediately give a negative reaction to warn you off. The same happens with smoking. If you give a cigarette to a non-smoker it will send them coughing, disoriented and dizzy. In some cases, it will make the person violently physically sick. This happens because the body naturally expels what it deems to be *foreign invaders*, or poisons, if you will. However, if the body thinks you have no choice but to have these *foreign invaders* coming in consistently, it will do what it can to negate the potential harmful effects and start building up an immunity and tolerance to them. This is why, and I know this from personal experience, having been a 2-3 packets of a cigarettes a day smoker, if you give a cigarette to a smoker it won't send them coughing, disorientated, dizzy or make them violently physically sick. This is because the smoker has built up an immunity and tolerance to the drug. Oddly, if you give a cigarette to a smoker who is coughing due to 'smoker's cough', they will more than likely stop coughing when they have the cigarette. This due to the hairs in the throat and lungs, called cilia. These hairs are supposed to be alive and well and are there to help to expel poisons from your lungs. When a heavy smoker goes to sleep, the hairs come alive and they often wake up with a 'smoker's cough'. This is the body doing what it's designed to do in order to expel the poisons and keep them as well as possible. If the smoker lights a cigarette, the smoke flattens the hairs and the person stops coughing – but this isn't a good thing. Equally, when you have been super clean on *Super Blend Me!* for a period of time, your system is much more attuned and sensitive to any foreign invaders – like a family sized bucket of KFC! This is why it is so important, after a set period of time on *nothing but Super Blends*, not to overburden your system with huge amounts of solid food, especially if it's refined or heavily processed. This doesn't mean you will be in pain if you grab a coffee and a biscuit, it just means you need to be a little more conscious of the fact that your stomach may have shrunk slightly and that your metabolism may also take a couple of days to get back to normal speed. You also need to be aware that your newly cleaned system may be more sensitive to overeating and *foreign invaders* than before your *Super Blend Me! Challenge.* However, none of this is an issue, as after a few days of gradually easing your body back onto good, clean, solid food, your stomach and metabolism will both return to their natural place.

RESETTING YOUR NATURAL CRAVINGS

Having said all of that, if you're like the vast majority of people who complete a *Super Blend Me! Challenge*, not only will a KFC be the last thing on your mind, but you should find you're actually *craving* healthy food. There is no question that most people, especially those doing longer than a 7-day *Super Blend Me! Challenge*, will end up craving solid food of some kind *before* their challenge ends. This is often more down to just wanting to sit and enjoy a meal that requires a knife and fork, rather than anything else. However, the foods people tend to crave most are usually things like an avocado or chicken salad, or a nice piece of hot salmon on a bed of rice – definitely **not** a McDonald's burger, fries and a Coke! This is because when you stop consuming refined sugars and fats, the body tends to stop craving refined sugars and fats. If you are reading this on your final day of your *Super Blend Me! Challenge* (as instructed) you'll know that what I am saying here is true. Your system seems to reset itself somehow, so you naturally crave good food. Your body, instinctively, has always craved good, nutritious food – it's your *mind* which overrides it and craves the crap. This is because of a combination of mind and chemical manipulation by BIG FOOD companies. It is in their financial interest for you to eat more of their product (so you buy more) which is why they try to make it as moreish and addictive as possible. They add just the right amounts of refined sugars, salts and fats to mess with your brain and confuse the body. They create 'food' in laboratories, which has been designed to have you coming back for more – and more often. For example, there are only so many apples you can eat, but that doesn't seem to apply to Pringles (they even tell you that 'once you pop, you can't stop').

Most of these foods are nutritionally empty and designed only to leave a person with a very frequent desire to top up their sugar levels, (which only dropped due to the last junk food 'fix'). It is a junk food merry-go-round that millions of people are on, but one that is actually pretty easy to get off. The good news is, having completed your *Super Blend Me! Challenge*, biochemistry-wise, you've already jumped off it. After a set period without refined sugars, fats or salts, your body should be wanting the good stuff.

Hopefully another thing you've realised from being on the *Super Blend Me! Challenge* is that we don't actually require huge amounts of food every day – we just need the *right* food every day. When it comes to nutrition, it's all about the quality of what is going in, rather than the quantity. Get the quality right, you instantly feel more *genuinely* satisfied, so your overall intake is naturally lowered. This is the key to lifelong success in this area – making sure you get *good quality* foods going into you, most of the time.

This, unfortunately, is easier said than done in today's nutritionally confusing world. It's not that most of us don't have access to a plethora of nutritious foods and drinks, we often just don't know which ones to pick. Not because we're stupid, but because everyone seems to have differing opinions as to what we should be eating, for optimum health. Even the 'experts' have opposing views, so how on earth is the layperson meant to know what to do? Chances are, this isn't the first book you've ever read on this subject, in which case you will know first-hand just how contradictory and confusing these messages can be.

One minute butter is the devil and margarine is the best thing since, and on, sliced bread. Then we hear margarine is about a molecule away from plastic and revert back to butter. One study says eggs are great, and another says more than three a week will give you a heart attack. We were told animal protein was off the table, now they're telling us it's back on – and don't get me started on fat! We were all told, with utter certainty, let's not forget, by just about every medical practitioner and 'qualified' dietician, that fat was the root of all dietary evil. This

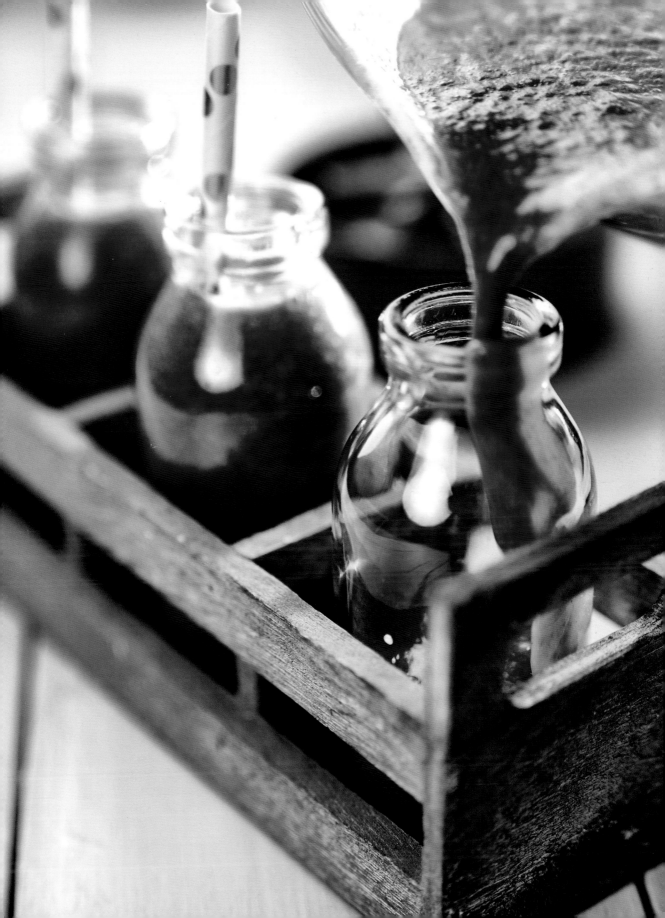

all stemmed from a study by Professor (no less), Ancel Keys. This guy was about as qualified as you can get, with PhDs from Berkeley and Cambridge, and an MSc just for good measure. It was his study 'proving' that fat is the major cause of heart disease and obesity which led to a fat-free frenzy. The fat-free mantra is only now just going away, as we realise that **fat** isn't in fact the major cause of heart disease and obesity that we were led to believe. Well, I say it's going away, but it's been hammered into us for so many decades that many are finding it hard to mentally release themselves from the 'fat is bad' grasp. It's now **sugar** that is the evil, and all sugar is now coming under attack! I once wrote an article with the headline *The Sugar In An Apple Is Not The Same As The Sugar In A Donut*. Even as I wrote it I wondered why I was even having to; after all, isn't this instinctively obvious? The problem is, when someone in a white coat, with 'scientifically backed' information spouts utter nonsense, people immediately believe it. This, of course, only goes on to confuse people even more! My conclusion to all of the confusing scientific studies by professors, conflicting what other equally qualified scientific professors are saying, is to strip it all down and simplify everything.

THERE'S ALWAYS ANOTHER WAY!

To that end, in this *Life After Super Blend Me!* section, you won't find a detailed list of permitted foods and drinks, but rather a common sense approach to healthy eating, which essentially puts all the power in your hands. Please don't be daunted by this; in fact, you should be excited to design a plan of your own which fits into *your* lifestyle, rather than having to follow someone else's specific diet. Clearly, if after you've read this book you decide to jump straight onto my *Super Food Me!* 7-Day Plan, for example, or perhaps my 5:2 *Juice Diet* (details coming up) then that's fine too. If you do either after you've read everything, then this will be your genuine choice and you won't be blindly following something just because there's no other option. Most people, unless they have a bigger health goal, usually embrace my 2:3:2 *Super Blend System* as a permanent way of life (coming up, so stay tuned!). However, even when people follow this lifestyle, they still effectively design their own 'diet'. What a person consumes on the 2:3:2 *Super Blend System* is largely down to the individual and they get to effectively design their own unique version of it.

The 2:3:2 *Super Blend System* is exactly what I live by, and it means I can be 'human' as well as healthy. It also doesn't matter if you're vegan, vegetarian, pescatarian or a meat eater – *everyone* can embrace their own version of this system which, when it comes to keeping the weight off, staying healthy and actually having a life, is perhaps the best I have experienced. However, before we get onto the *Life After Super Blend Me!* section, let's continue with the 'simplifying everything' theme.

GO 'NO LABEL'!

For years, I was asked over and over again by people concerned about their health, 'What am I looking for on the label?' It took me many years to realise that the problem was the label itself and so now, whenever people ask me, 'What am I looking for on the label?', I simply reply, **'THE LABEL!'**

Fruits, vegetables, grains, nuts, seeds and lean proteins don't require a label and these are the very foods we need to be consuming the vast majority of the time to stay lean and healthy. It's not even something we need a lesson in; we all know instinctively what is meant by *No Label* food. It's the only food all wild animals consume and we would naturally be drawn to if BIG FOOD hadn't manipulated and chemicalized our food. It is also the food that you should be naturally drawn to, now you have completed your *Super Blend Me! Challenge*. Your system is now clean and, like I mentioned earlier, any junk food addiction should have subsided and you should now be naturally craving nutritious, *No Label* foods.

AVOID ALL MYSTERY FOOD!

Despite having incredibly strict food label laws, it appears that the same strict rules don't apply to *mystery food*. You may not be familiar with this term, that's because I made it up! It seems astonishing that things like hot dogs at a cinema or burgers served by a very large dribbly man, from a greasy burger van outside a nightclub, don't require a label (or even an ingredients list for that matter). This is good news for the seller, because if people actually knew what was in their 'food', I'm unsure they'd make any sales. Clearly, it's bad news for the consumer, as what they're eating remains a mystery. I suppose you could argue that technically, these foods are also *No Label*, but obviously not in keeping with the *No Label* diet principles I am talking about here. This is why I put them under a completely separate category – *mystery food*. It's funny how when you see the dribbly burger van man before going into a nightclub you think, *how can anyone eat that rubbish?*, but then a few drinks later you're queuing up at 2am to get hold of some… such is the mind bending power of alcohol! I would advise steering clear of mystery food at **all** times, and, if you're a drinker, you may want to relax a little on that front too.

WATCH OUT FOR THE CLASSIC 'HEALTHY HEADLINE' LABEL TRICKS!

If you do find yourself drawn to the often inviting 'healthy headlines' on some foods and drinks, think twice before buying into them. BIG FOOD will use anything at their disposal to try and spin their product in a *healthy* direction. They will use everything from the classic *Fat-Free* and *Sugar-Free* headlines, to putting pictures of fields all over their packaging in a bid to convince you that their product is all natural. Tesco, a large UK supermarket chain, is even allowed to use *Farm Foods* as a brand name on their packets, even though the food never originated from a farm. They had *Rosedene Farms* on things like apples, pears, strawberries and blueberries; *Willow Farms* on chicken, and *Boswell Farms* on beef products. Not only did these foods never generate from cute little farms, but these particular farms are completely made up – they simply don't exist! Tesco, of course, are far from the only, what I describe as, *healthy headline* tricksters, most BIG FOOD companies are at it. They will use pictures of green fields, healthy looking people and, as we know, pay huge sums of money to top athletes to

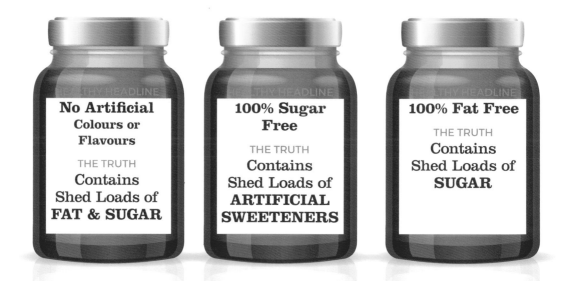

No Artificial
Colours or
Flavours

THE TRUTH
Contains
Shed Loads of
FAT & SUGAR

100% Sugar
Free

THE TRUTH
Contains
Shed Loads of
ARTIFICIAL
SWEETENERS

100% Fat Free

THE TRUTH
Contains
Shed Loads of
SUGAR

promote their product and give the impression that their body and gold medal was down to that particular food or drink. I don't have time here to go through all the tricks, (labels on their own could be an entire book) but I thought I'd include the classics and then give their real meaning, just so you're armed!

These are the most commonly used, but equally don't be fooled by terms like *fair-trade, organic, gluten-free, wheat-free* and so on. The second we see something that's organic and fair trade we think it's healthy. But I can get hold of some very premium fair trade, organic, sugar-free, fat-free, gluten-free, wheat-free and artificial-sweetener-free...cocaine! If you have a 40% refined sugar, fair trade, organic bar, it's still not good just because of the *fair trade* and *organic* status. It would be slightly healthier and clearly more ethical, but it's still not healthy with 40% white refined sugar in.

CAN YOU FIND IT ON AN ISLAND?

No Label is an incredibly simple way to instantly recognise if a food or drink is healthier than the next. However, there is another term that I also really like, that comes from non-other than Jon Gabriel (he's the guy who dropped over 200lbs eating *No Label* foods and drinking *No Label* juices). Jon eats and drinks by a very similar principle to *No Label* and has one question for the people he coaches to eat well: 'Can you find it on an island?' If you can find it on an island, then you are good to go. If you can grow it, fish it or hunt it – it's *No Label* and the body will recognise it. You cannot, for example, find MSG (**M**ono**s**odium **G**lutamate) or HFCS (**H**igh **F**ructose **C**orn **S**yrup) on an island, so they are definite no gos!

IT'S ALL ABOUT LOW H.I. FOODS AND DRINKS!

In terms of further simplification this is, in my opinion, the *easiest* and best approach to diet I have ever come across. I personally no longer use the term *No Label* and I can't find everything I want to eat on an Island – so instead I apply a *Low H.I.* principle to the *vast majority* of what I eat and drink. Like *No Label, Low H.I.* is not only incredibly easy to understand and almost impossible to argue against, but it also takes away the majority of dietary confusion. *Low H.I.* stands for **L**ow **H**uman **I**ntervention; in other words, no matter what the food or drink, all you are looking for is how much a human has interfered with it. The more it's been interfered with, the worse it tends to be – simple. An orange picked directly from a tree, for example, is *No H.I.,* and something like a heavily processed, refined sugar and fat-laced muffin is *High H.I.* We need to understand that only wild animals eat nothing but *No H.I.* foods, and in order for us to do the same, we'd also have to live in the wild and have skills like Bear Grylls in order to survive. Luckily we don't need to eat *No H.I.* in order to be slim and healthy, as the body can deal with a *certain amount* of just about *anything* and still stay healthy. We have a truly incredible inbuilt filtration system, which can deal with all sorts of crap and still keep you in fine fettle. This amazing filtration system is the reason why, after smoking 2-3 packets of cigarettes a day for years, drinking shedloads of alcohol on a daily basis, and eating crap from morning till night – I am still here! Clearly, if I had carried on, I honestly believe I wouldn't be here today, as the body can only deal with a certain amount of rubbish, not the bucketloads I was pouring in. What this illustrates is that if you have a cheeky flat white or piece of carrot cake, for example, you won't get ill or die! However, we do need to make sure that the *vast majority* of what goes into our body is *Low H.I.* in order for the filtration system to work efficiently, and in order for us to have the luxury of 'being human' with no adverse effects. This is why the *2:3:2 Super Blend System* is so effective, as it meets these needs perfectly (don't worry, it's coming!)

IT DOESN'T MATTER IF YOU ARE A VEGAN, VEGGIE, PESCI OR MEAT EATER - LOW H.I. WORKS FOR ALL!

Again, what I really love about the *Low H.I.* way of life is that it doesn't matter if you're a vegetarian, vegan or otherwise – *Low H.I.* applies to any *No Label* foods such as fruits, vegetables, grains, nuts, seeds, and lean proteins. This gets rid of the usual nutritional arguments which can take up days of your life, such as whether you should eat meat or have dairy. My mission is not to turn anyone into a vegetarian or vegan. If you choose to go down that route feel free. Equally, if you don't think vegetarianism or veganism is for you, don't become one. The key behind the *Low H.I.* way of eating and drinking is simply to think about what you are about to consume and ask yourself, 'Is it *Low H.I.?*'

If you are going to eat meat at least make sure it's *Low H.I.*, for your sake and, of course, the sake of the animals. Ask yourself, Was it reared organically and did it have natural food throughout its life?' If that's the case, it's *Low H.I.*, if not, it isn't. If you're eating honey, is it *Low H.I.*? Some honey has been interfered with so much by humans, that it's no longer a natural *Low H.I.* sweetener, but more a *High H.I.* locally grown version of honey; as close to what nature intended honey is what you're looking for. If you're going to have milk, then is it from an organic, grass-fed dairy cow? With *Low H.I.* nothing is out of bounds, as long as it's a *Low H.I.* version. Bread is a really good example of just how far removed from nature a food product can get. You can get bad very *High H.I.* bread and good *Low H.I.* bread and in terms of nutrition, they are worlds apart from each other. Most of the bread on sale in supermarkets is loaded with sugar and chemicals and is nothing more than sugar in your bloodstream (and a bloated lump in your stomach). However, flat breads like pumpernickel and German rye bread are *Low H.I.* and therefore a much better option. You are looking for the closest to the grain as possible, and where humans have interfered the least.

If you do eat meat then always ask yourself, 'Is it at least *Low H.I.*?' In other words, is the chicken free range and organic, or is it one dose of chemicals away from a science experiment? If you eat fish, is it *Low H.I.*? Does it look like a piece of fish or is it a bunch of fish parts from lots of different fish disguised in breadcrumbs? If you are eating tomatoes, are they organic and do they at least look like nice, dark, ripe tomatoes, or just a load of squashed chemical-rich tomatoes that have been mixed with sugar and other junk to form a ketchup?

I could give a million examples, but the beauty of *Low H.I.* living is that it is pretty much self-explanatory. There will be some people out there who want to follow a *No H.I.* diet. *No H.I.* living is clearly where you pick an apple from the tree yourself, from an organic field. This is just a little too much to ask for the average person, and as far as I'm concerned, life's too short. You don't, after all, want to spend your one and only life trying to extend your life, only to miss it in the process, because that is all you focused on! There clearly needs to be a balance, but again it's the ratio of that balance that is important. *High H.I.* living is where all you eat is junk, where everything has been massively processed and interfered with. This is why a *Low H.I.* way of life is the best of all worlds. You are simply looking for foods and drinks that have had *some* human intervention, but not enough to destroy the nutrients or to have added nasties which could cause you harm.

YOU DON'T WANT TO SPEND YOUR ONE AND ONLY LIFE TRYING TO EXTEND YOUR LIFE ONLY TO REALISE YOU MISSED YOUR LIFE IN THE PROCESS!

Here's a quick overview of the *Low H.I.* or *No Label* (if you prefer) way of life. Once again, this is not set in stone, nor is it scientific, but it's a good common sense guideline and it's up to you to ultimately design your own diet so that you are not on a diet.

THE LOW H.I. WAY OF LIFE

50% Fruits & Vegetables in the form of blends, juices, soups and salads, etc.

25% Proteins such as *Low H.I.* fish, meat, nuts, seeds, etc.

15% Good Grains such as rice, whole rye, quinoa, oats, buckwheat, millet, bulgur wheat, etc.

10% Junk Food *High H.I.* foods and drinks.

Usually, after the *Super Blend Me! Challenge*, many people avoid all *High H.I.* foods and drinks because they feel so good and clearly you aren't obligated to have the 10% *High H.I.* The reason I have factored it into the equation is for two fundamental reasons:

1. We need to understand, and I really don't mind repeating this point to hammer it home, the body can deal with a certain amount of anything without experiencing any weight gain or illness. I was extremely strict for many years and was, for want of a better phrase, a right royal pain in the arse (or *ass* for my American readers). Friends stopped inviting me for dinner in the end as I was obsessed with food and was always trying to do the right thing. I wasn't eating any junk at all and was on a 100% *Low H.I.* diet, 100% of the time. I thought by not eating any junk I had removed my food problem, but all I had done, to some

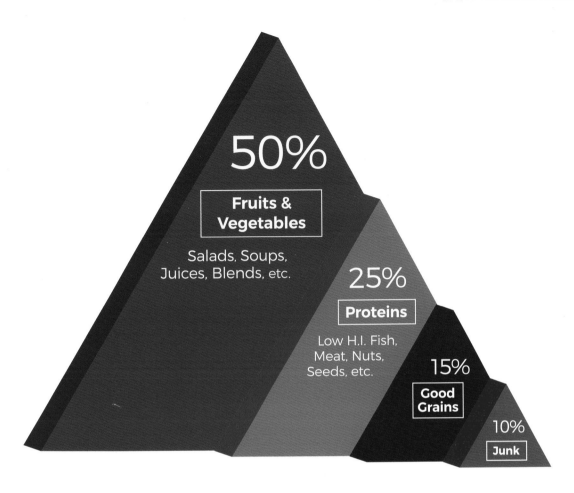

extent at least, was *move* it, not *remove* it. Freedom is about choice and being able to design your own diet without becoming obsessed. We need to give our body some credit; it was designed to deal with a certain amount of anything. That certain amount however, is about 10% maximum of what you eat in a day. This rule clearly goes out the window if you go to Vegas for a week! (Come on, you're in Vegas!).

2. We are human! And as humans we have dinner parties and, if we want a life with our friends and family, we need to not be anal about food. Food is fuel and it is vital that the vast majority of fuel going into the body is the fuel designed to run it efficiently (*Low H.I. living*). At the same time, because we are human, it is also important to be free to have some *High H.I.* foods and drinks, if the occasion calls for it. If your little one has made some cakes, you don't want to say, 'Sorry I only eat *Low H.I.*!'

Some of you may want to continue on a blend-only way of life for a few more days, or even weeks, after you finish your initial *Super Blend Me! Challenge*. The choice is yours and clearly you can do what you like, you can even go and eat rubbish from here on in, but why would you want to throw away what you've already achieved? Just focus on how amazing you feel right now – why would you ever want to go back?

IT IS POSSIBLE TO HAVE TOO MUCH OF A GOOD THING!

As crazy as this sounds, it's true, and it also applies to good food. We only need a certain amount of food / fuel each day and that differs greatly from person to person and the level of physical activity they take on. This is why I covered this fully in the *7 Rules For Success* before you started your challenge. I didn't want you forcing yourself to drink all of your *Super Blends* if your body clearly didn't want them. Many people think, as long as it's healthy, it doesn't matter how much they consume. The area I have seen this way of thinking to be most prominent is in the raw food world. As the name suggests, 'raw fooders' eat nothing but raw food and are usually vegans (although not always). They never heat their food above a certain temperature and everything must be, well, raw. You would think, therefore, that their main diet would consist of large avocado salads and plates of vegetables. However, this isn't always the case. Many miss cooked food greatly and sugar even more. This is why they will often eat shedloads of nuts and find whatever sugar alternative they can get their hands on to get their 'fix'. Agave nectar was the sugar substitute of choice for years, but in real terms, it's almost as bad as actual white refined sugar. Many raw fooders eat huge raw desserts and wonder why they are still fat and sick. However, even if you are skipping the agave nectar and eating extremely well, the sheer *amount* you eat will always play a huge role in your health and weight. This is why, of all the rules to follow, one of the most important, *especially* when eating food, is...

The
JAPANESE
RULE

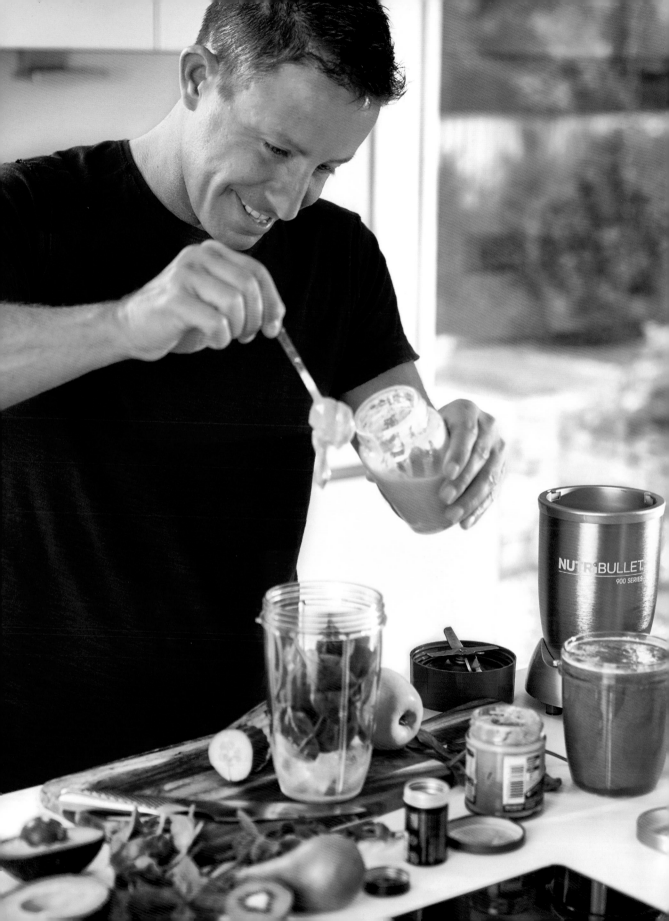

There is a principle in personal development known as 'modeling'. This is where, instead of looking to reinvent the wheel, you find someone who is already getting the success you want in a certain area (so health and weight loss, in this case) and you simply model them. In other words, do what they are doing and you should reap the same rewards.

With the *Japanese Rule* you can go much further and model an entire nation. There are flaws in modeling just one person, as individual people can have different results to another individual, but if you look at Japanese people as a nation, they're worth modeling on the health front. A recent study showed that the Japanese have the longest life expectancy, for both men and women, and the least amount of degenerative diseases, compared to any other nation on earth. To put some perspective on this, men in the US were ranked 29th in the world and US women 33rd! This is even more ironic when you think about it, as the US spends over $2.7 trillion *annually* on health care. This is worth repeating and in capitals and bold so it really registers:

THE US SPENDS OVER $2.7 TRILLION ANNUALLY ON HEALTH CARE

The UK didn't make it into the top ten either, despite the billions spent on the NHS. The researchers involved in the study believed it was diet, above all else, which had the largest bearing on the statistics. They looked at their intake of omega-3 rich foods and also fermented foods and came to the conclusion that these must play a large part in their health and longevity success. Now, I have no doubt that *what* they eat plays a massive role in why they live so long, disease free, but I also feel an even more important clue lies in *how* they eat.

HARA HACHI BU

The Japanese live by an eating principle known as *hara hachi bu*, a phrase which roughly translates to, 'eat until you are eight parts full', or 'belly 80% full'. As of the early 21st century, Okinawans in Japan, through practicing *hara hachi bu*, are the only human population to have a self-imposed habit of calorie restriction. On average, they consume 1,800 – 1,900 calories a day and have the highest concentration of centenarians (people over the age of 100) on earth.

"EIGHT PARTS OF A FULL STOMACH SUSTAIN THE MAN; THE OTHER TWO SUSTAIN THE DOCTOR."
Hakuun Yasutani

I'm not a big 'calorie' person as you know, and I feel a great deal of the calorie model is flawed, as it's about the *quality* of the calorie, not simply the calorie itself. However, a great deal of research has been done on food restriction and has shown time and time again an increase in life expectancy. So, if you are a big eater, the message is clear: eat a little less now, you'll live longer and therefore ultimately get to eat a lot more!

By applying, what I term as the *Japanese Rule* of *hara hachi bu* to whatever you eat will go a long way to keeping you on the road to optimum health. This is why I was so adamant in *Rule 3* (page??) about drinking your blends slowly and only until satisfied. It is extremely important, even with good food (or blends) that you never force in more than the body wants. What you eat is clearly important, and *Low H.I.* is the way to go wherever you can, but how you eat is just as important. However, it is much easier to apply the *Japanese Rule* of *hara hachi bu* to *Low H.I.* foods than *High H.I.* foods. *High H.I.* foods, containing loads of refined fat, salt and sugar, are often created in a laboratory and are designed to be addictive and have no natural 'cut off' point. The chocolate Hobnob biscuit perhaps sums it up best with their advertising slogan, *One Nibble and You're Nobbled!* It is much easier to leave the table at 80% full if you've been eating fish and salad, but near to impossible after fish and chips. Natural food, or *Low H.I. / Super / No Label /Found on an Island*, or however you like to term it, doesn't cause a disproportionate surge in insulin production. It is only when insulin levels are lowered that a person can feel satisfied, which is the main reason why the *Japanese Rule* is much easier to apply with *Low H.I.* foods than *High H.I.* foods. *Low H.I.* food doesn't tend to cause a sudden spike in blood sugar with the knock-on effect of increased insulin production; *High H.I.*, on the other hand, does tend to.

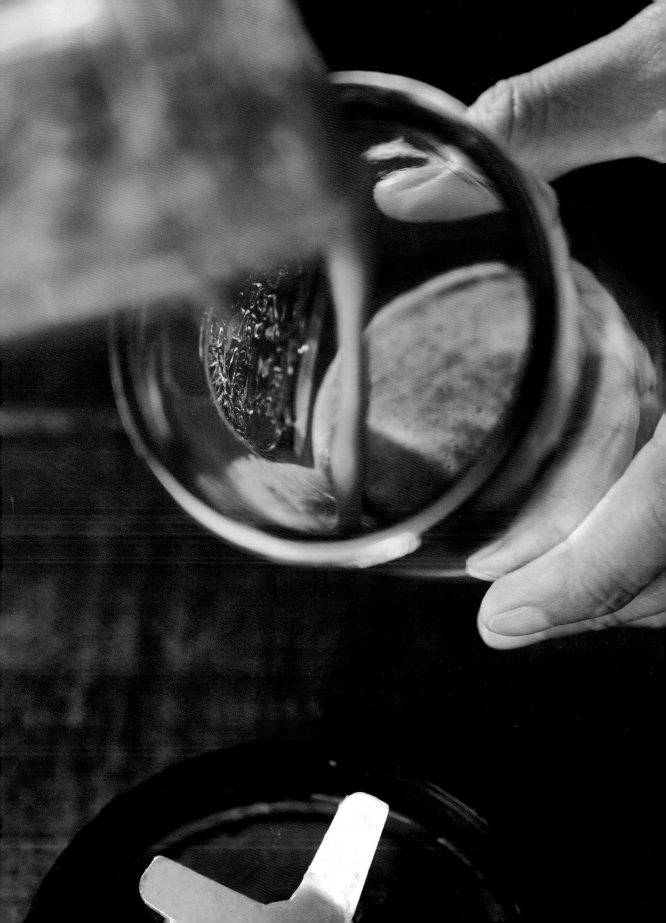

There will, of course, be times when you eat *High H.I.* here and there, but you can still adopt the *Japanese Rule*. Yes, it may be more of a challenge, but if you reach about 80% full, wait 20 minutes, by which time you tend to feel 100% full. It usually only takes about 20 minutes for the signals to go from the stomach to the brain and for the insulin levels to be lowered. Even if, for whatever reason, you go back to eating crap (and I sincerely hope you don't) at least give yourself a fighting chance by adopting the *Japanese Rule* for life. Apply this principle on top of a *Low H.I.* majority diet, and you'll be doing exactly what it takes to maintain a healthy and lean body. But please, please, please remember to also be human!

Right, now we've stripped away the confusion and you're armed with the basic principles, we can finally take a look at where you might venture on the food front after your *Super Blend Me! Challenge*. As I mentioned, you can either design your own plan or simply jump directly onto one I have laid out for you, it's your call, but before you decide, make a point of reading the five follow-on options I have laid out in...

5
CHEEKY
ways to stay on
TRACK

FOR YOUR CONSIDERATION

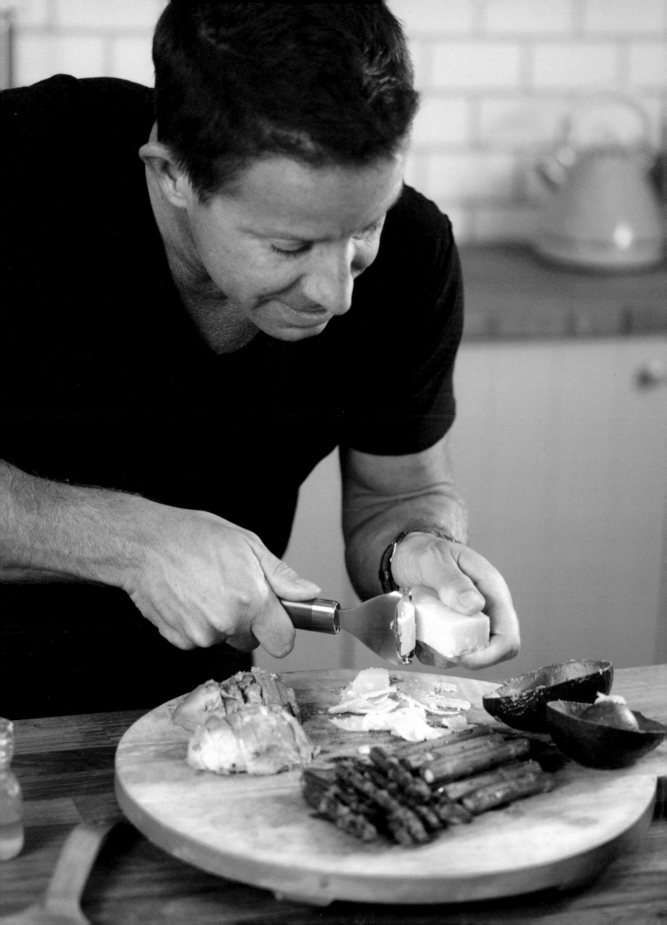

OPTION 1

THE 2-3-2 SUPER BLEND SYSTEM

I have added this one first as it's the system I personally live by and the one I most highly recommend. This is the perfect follow-on plan for anyone who wishes to keep their weight and health in check, but at the same time wants the freedom to be human!

I think it's naive to think that just because you've done a week (or more) on nothing but *Super Blends*, that you're going to be cleaner than clean for the rest of your life. You might well be one of the few who are, but most wish to opt for a 'nutrition for reality' approach. If you do have a lot more weight to lose, or you really need to get your health on track, then you may well be super clean, or even continue on *Super Blends*, until you reach your health and weight goals. However, once you have arrived at that place you may feel the human need to be, well, more human! We are looking for something that works on every level, and for me, this works a treat and means I can actually live in the normal human world and have friends, too!

The principles of the *2-3-2 System* are quite simple:

2 DAYS A WEEK ON BLENDS OR JUICE
3 DAYS LOW H.I. LIVING
2 DAYS ON ANYTHING YOU LIKE!

My two days on pure juices / blends tend to consist of either four juices a day, or a blend for breakfast and then two or three fresh juices throughout the day. However, I am conscious that for most reading this, *Super Blends* will be your preference. Most are attracted to *Super Blend Me!* because it means they don't have to clean a juicer, so if this was one of your motivations for taking on the challenge, I am guessing you're now hooked and, if you choose the *2-3-2 System*, you'll opt for

Super Blends rather than juices. If you are having juices, you can have up to four a day, but with blends – because they have a slightly higher calorie count – you only need three. I don't usually do the calorie thing, but here it's relevant as the two days on pure juices / blends is based around the principles of the famous 5:2 *Diet*. In the original 5:2 *Diet*, the advice was to have a maximum of 600 calories for two days a week, and eat whatever you want for the remaining five days. The problem with this diet was twofold:

1. On the two days of 600 calories, it didn't matter where you got those calories.

2. Five days a week you were told you could eat anything.

You could follow this and have zero live nutrition going into your body – ever! I also know people who would stuff themselves senseless for five days a week, believing the two days on 600 calories would negate any damage done. This clearly isn't the case, and you'd be amazed at the damage you can do in five days, especially if you're doing that every week. For those who only eat crap, then the 5:2 *Diet* does them good. They effectively get involved with some scientifically backed up intermittent fasting for two days a week, and therefore will be better off than they would have been had they stuffed themselves for seven days rather than five. There are, of course, some who do the 5:2 *Diet* intelligently and don't eat like a horse on the non-fasting days, but many do, and it's why I encourage my *2-3-2 System* with some clear guidelines for the majority of non-fasting days. Clearly, if you do have three blends a day, it would be around 1,000 calories, not the 600 as studied in the 5:2 principles. However, if you want to stick strictly to roughly 600 calories a day, then it would be two *Super Blends*. Having said that, I have found anything between 600-1,000 calories achieves similar results, especially if you are exercising as well. Once again though, don't get too caught up in obsessive calorie counting, life's too short!

The good news is, having just spent a significant length of time on three *Super Blends* a day for the duration of your challenge, doing just two days a week will seem like an absolute breeze.

You can also play the *2-3-2 System* how you like, as you don't have to do the two *juice / blend only* days consecutively. My week changes all the time depending on my diary commitments. Sometimes I have a *juice / blend only* day on a Monday and Wednesday, other times it's a Wednesday and Thursday. However, one thing is for sure, virtually each and every week, for two days, I'm on pure juices / blends. I then eat mainly from my *Super fast Food* book for three days – still having a juice or blend first thing – and then for two days a week I have no set rules at all. This system has allowed me to not only fully maintain my weight and general health, but it means I get to have friends and a life too! As mentioned, I was *extremely* clean for many years and, although I felt great, the only people who wanted to hang out with me were other extremely clean people (and trust me, not all extremely clean people are the most fun people to hang out with!). The two 'human' days are when you'll see me grabbing a flat white, eating things you wouldn't expect and, on occasions, you may even see me sipping a cheeky glass of champagne. I don't always choose the weekends as human days, either; flexibility is always the key to feeling free, and freedom is what it's all about. Whenever I'm at an airport, I'll have whatever I fancy, and will always make an airport day a human day and then adjust the week accordingly. The *2-3-2 System* is explained fully in my *5:2 Juice Diet* book, but here's a rough idea of what your version might look like:

Mon / Tue:

4x juices **or** 3x *Super Blends* a day

Wed / Thu / Fri:

Low H.I. meals, usually consisting of a juice or blend for breakfast, a nice fresh salad for lunch, and one of the lovely dinners from the *Super fast Food* book / app.

Sat / Sun:

Whatever you like! This, funnily enough, usually still consists of a juice or blend for breakfast (because you are so used to it and will almost crave it); a lunch consisting of anything with no rules; and the same for dinner. It's also the two days where, if you do like a glass or two of wine, you can have it. You then clean up again on Monday and Tuesday, balance out on Wednesday, Thursday, Friday, and enjoy the weekend with your friends, however you see fit.

The key is, **DON'T BE RIGID**. It is extremely important that if you do choose this particular follow-on system, it becomes what you do *most* of the time – but maybe not all the time. You have to be open to life's rich tapestry, so be flexible and let common sense prevail.

OPTION 2

SUPER FOOD ME! 7-DAY PLAN

This is taken from my *Super fast food* book / app and there are two 7-day plans to choose from; one vegetarian and one pescatarian. Each day starts with a blend, but feel free to swap those recipes for any of the *Super Blend* you have come to love on your *Super Blend Me! Challenge*.

The *Super fast Food* book and app feature all the recipes for both plans, as well as a shopping list for the entire seven days. The app goes one stage further and will even auto-generate a shopping list for however many days you want to shop for. If you wish to devise your own specific follow-on meal plan from the recipes in the app (of which there are over 100) then clearly feel free. The app makes this super-easy as you can simply select what you want for breakfast, lunch and dinner and again, it will auto-generate a shopping list for you, for however many days you wish to shop for. Many who choose to design their own plan after their *Super Blend Me! Challenge* often choose either a lunch and dinner, or just a dinner, from *Super fast Food*. This is because most are in such a groove that they often continue with *Super Blends* for breakfast and lunch, even after they have finished the challenge itself. There are many who will choose the *2-3-2 System* and will use the recipes from the book / app to fit around their own version of it.

If you do choose to follow one of the *Super Food Me!* 7-day plans, afterwards, you may still choose to continue using recipes from the book / app as they are all perfectly balanced and adhere to the *Low H.I.* way of life beautifully. Actually, I nearly named that book the *Low H.I.* Cookbook, but unless you know what *Low H.I.* really means, it wouldn't have made any sense. I also nearly called it *There's More To Life Than Quinoa*, because there is! There isn't a classic dish you can't put a healthy twist on, including fish 'n' chips, burger and fries, and a curry (all of which can be found in the *Super fast Food* book / app).

OPTION 3

THE BBM PLAN

Usually, by the time you finish your *Super Blend Me! Challenge*, you are so used to having a blend for breakfast and lunch that many simply continue this. The *BBM* plan, isn't so much a plan, but rather a way of life that a lot of people automatically move towards when the main challenge is done. *BBM* is **B**LEND / **B**LEND / **M**EAL and is pretty much how I live for 4 / 5 days a week. Although I have two days a week on pure juice or blends as part of the *2-3-2 System*, I often just have either juices or blends throughout the day on *Low H.I.* days too. *BBM* is also the perfect option for those who really have no desire to spend two days a week on nothing but blends, yet don't mind the idea of having *Super Blends* throughout the day, providing they can use their teeth in the evening. Clearly you can adapt and make it *JJM* (**J**uice / **J**uice / **M**eal) if you are more into those, but as you have just done *Super Blend Me!* I'm guessing *BBM* will be more up your street. Remember, you choose whichever fruit and vegetable juices / blends you like for breakfast and lunch, and then eat in the evening – simples!

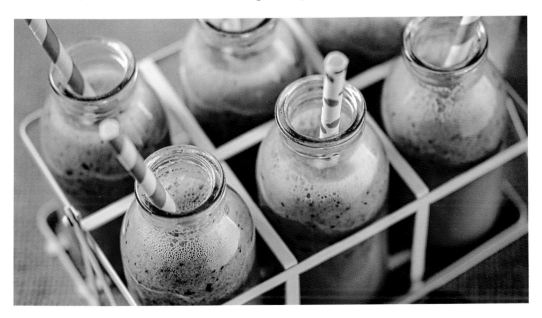

OPTION 4

THE BMM PLAN

I think you already know where I'm going with this one. It's **B**lend / **M**eal / **M**eal. However, the meals should clearly be *Low H.I.* where possible. Perhaps a juice/blend for breakfast, salad / soup for lunch and then whatever you fancy for dinner; usually a more substantial meal, like an avocado salad with a nice piece of fish, or whatever floats your *Low H.I.* boat. Many mix between the *BBM* and *BMM* way of life and it's usually enough to keep most in fine fettle.

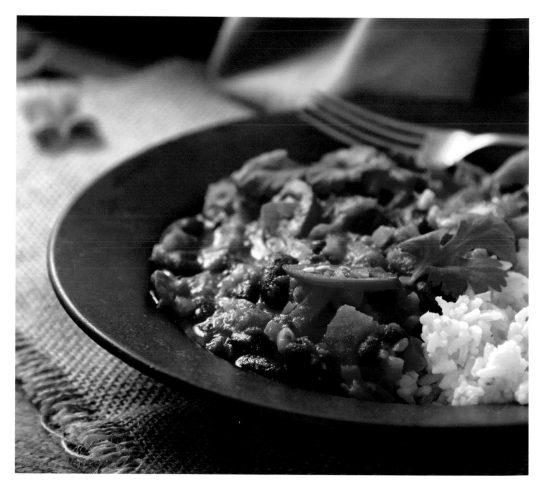

OPTION 5

2:5 SUPER BLEND ME! SYSTEM

This is the option for people who still have a significant amount of weight to lose / a significant health challenge they still need to overcome, and feel they can't continue on just *Super Blends*. The principles here are simple:

• 2 Days A Week On Good Food
• 5 Days A Week on Super Blends

There are some people who will simply extend their *Super Blend Me! Challenge* until they reach their goal, whilst others need to introduce some solid food into their world before they go nuts!

Having been in this industry for over two decades now, I am fully aware that there are many people who have an enormous amount of weight to lose and several health challenges to overcome due to their excess weight. Whilst I know that a prolonged period on pure *Super Blends* (sometimes months) would give them the best results in the shortest time, I am also aware that few could mentally do it. This is why I have included the option of the 2:5 *Super Blend Me!* System. This option means you have your whole weekend to enjoy some delicious yet nutritious food, whilst remaining on your journey to the land of the slim and healthy. I would still strongly advise that your two eating days are *good food* eating days, for two reasons:

1. It will mean you reach your goal faster.
2. It won't trigger addictions.

It's reason number two I wish to focus on here, as it's probably the *most* important. If you binge on nothing but junk on your two eating days, the following week will be much harder. Firstly, you'll have to deal with withdrawal again. If you remember back to the first two / three days of your *Super Blend Me! Challenge*, you may recall some headaches or drop in energy, so I'm guessing you really don't want to have to deal with that *every week* until you reach your goal? Secondly, and more importantly, you risk triggering the addiction part of life. Please never underestimate the invisible pull that white refined sugar, fat and salt can have on you – *especially* if you have been addicted before. If you choose this option, it means you are on a significant journey and you want to make it as easy as possible. Eating junk for two days a week **will not** give you respite from cravings, it will simply trigger *more* of them, making your journey far more challenging than it needs to be. My advice couldn't be stronger on this one . . .

EAT GOOD FOOD ON YOUR TWO EATING DAYS TO AVOID TRIGGERING ADDICTION AND WITHDRAWAL

That's almost it folks, just one final thing...

BLEND IT
FORWARD
et) help to make
A DIFFERENCE!

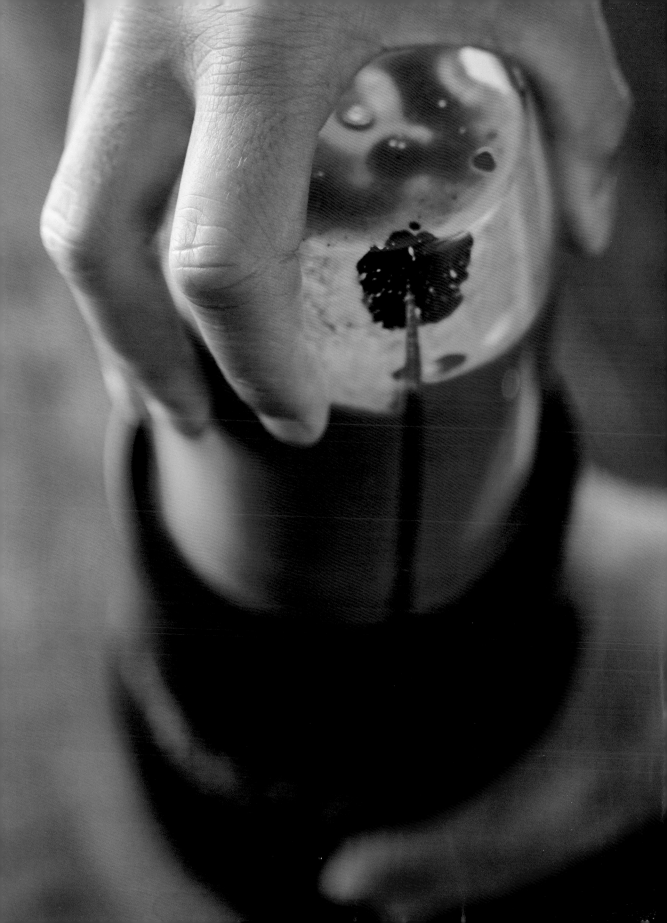

As I mentioned at the start of this book, I set out over 20 years ago to Juice The World. My mission was to make a juicer and blender as common as a kettle and a toaster in everyone's kitchen.

I also wanted to make sure these two potentially lifesaving pieces of kit would take pride of place on the kitchen work surface and not be relegated to 'cupboardsville' like the poor old breadmaker. Juicers and blenders are now prevalent in most kitchens, so my mission has now shifted slightly. I now not only want a juicer and blender to be as common as a kettle and a toaster, but I also want to make sure people use them...and use them *correctly*. This is one of the main driving forces behind this book. I frequently see people with bullet-type blenders either making blends containing more calories than a meal at a fast food joint, or what amounted to the consistency of a thick cold soup better served in a bowl than a glass! Like with my mission to *Juice The World*, my mission to get people using their healthy hardware correctly cannot be done by myself alone, and this is where you come in.

THROW A SUPER BLEND ME! PARTY

For a long time now I have encouraged people to throw a Super *Juice* Me! party. This is where people make a load of juices from that plan and play my movie of the same name. Clearly, I haven't made the movie Super *Blend* Me! yet (although it is coming, look out for it) so you can't throw a Super Blend Me! party. However, don't let that stop you from *Blending It Forward* and helping to make a difference. You could run a mini 'blending master class' for the many, *many* people who haven't got a clue when it comes to the right way to make a decent and easy to digest blend – after all, now you've done the plan you should be pretty up to speed on blending mastery! You could run through the *7 Rules* and *7 Tips For Success* or if you have the app, beam my videos onto a big screen while you all enjoy a blending taster session. You could also share all the results from people all over the world, or maybe it's just a case of you singing from the rooftops just how effective *Super Blend Me!* is and, in turn, organically inspiring your friends and family to try a challenge on for size. These days we have social media, which can be incredibly powerful in a positive way when used correctly. If you are on a few of the most used social media platforms, then sing about what you have achieved and help to make a huge difference out there. We have a *genuine* obesity and health crisis and even if your story helps just one person, then it has to be worth the few minutes it takes to share. If you want your inspiring results to reach more people, then send them to *results@superjuiceme.com* and we'll share your achievements with a much wider audience. Also, please make sure you tag me in: here are my social media channels again ,in case you missed them earlier:

Right, that really is it! Congratulations again on doing whatever it took to complete your personal *Super Blend Me! Challenge*, and if I don't bump into you at one of my seminars or retreats, continue to do whatever it takes to make your health a top priority in your life. There has never been a more truthful saying than, 'If you haven't got your health you've got nothing', so make health your new wealth and thank you in advance for helping to spread the message and inspire others.

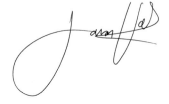

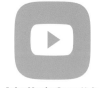

JuiceMasterJasonVale   JasonVale   JuiceMasterLtd   JuiceMaster

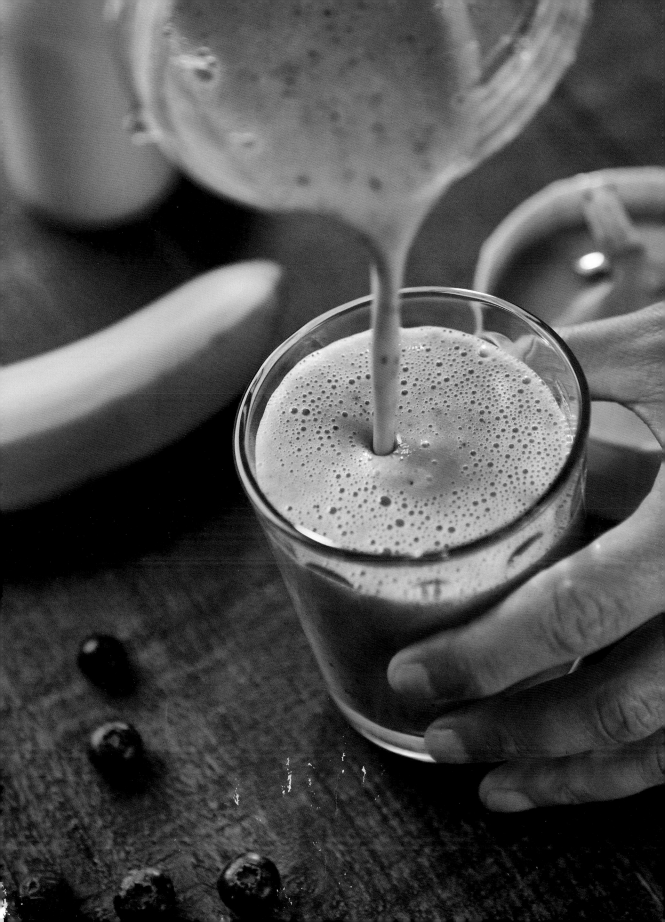

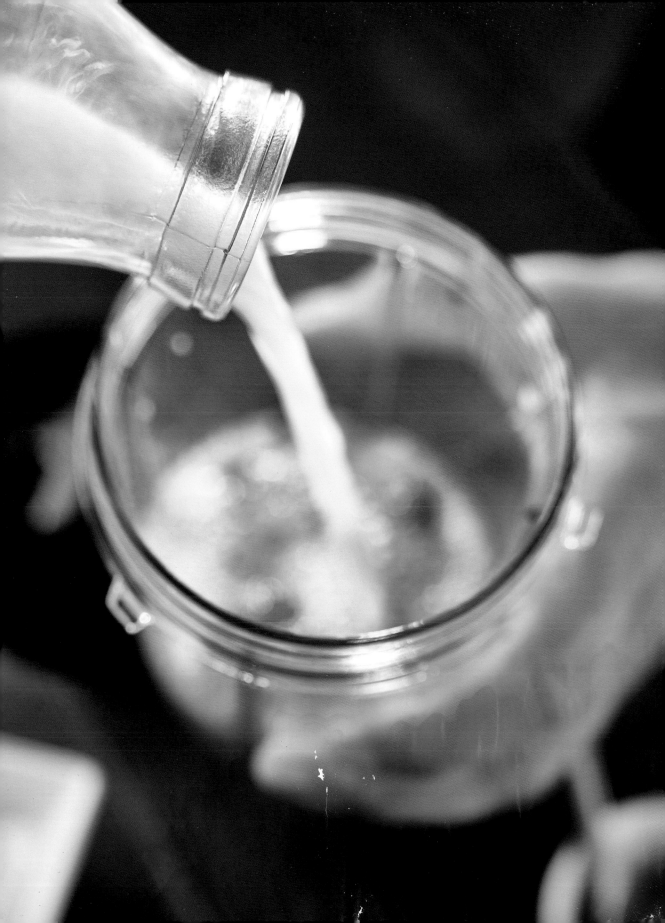

Q+A

Q. YOU ARE THE JUICE MASTER, IS THIS BLEND PLAN BETTER THAN YOUR JUICE PLANS?

A. Yes and no! If you are the type of person who would never do one of my *juice* plans due to having to clean a juicer, then yes, this *blend* plan is better than not doing a plan at all. However, if you are someone who would embrace one of my juice plans, then I would say *Super **Juice** Me!* is better than *Super **Blend** Me!*

The reason for this is due to the sheer level of micronutrients and plethora of ingredients that go into the *Super **Juice** Me!* plan. There are many things which are better juiced (such as raw beetroot, carrots, etc.) and mean the level of good quality, raw plant nutrition in *Super **Juice** Me!*, is higher than in *Super **Blend** Me!* The blends I have put together in the *Super **Juice** Me!* plan are a combination of freshly extracted juices, which are then blended with some avocado or banana. The blends in *Super **Blend** Me!* use the liquid from either coconut milk, coconut water, almond milk or oat milk. These are wonderful nutritious liquids, but, for me, don't match up to some freshly extracted organic vegetable juice as the liquid. That said, *Super **Blend** Me!* is actually better for some people, like those who are already pretty lean and wish to sustain the exercise they are doing, lose body fat and gain muscle mass. It also appeals to those people who simply don't have enough time to do a juice plan.

I personally now do both depending on my mood and goals. Sometimes, I'll have a blend for breakfast and lunch, other times I go back to my juices. I still feel the ultimate juice / blend combo is the *Turbo Charge Smoothie* from my *7-Day Juice Challenge*. I have made a blend only version of that recipe in this *Super Blend Me!* plan, but I still feel you can't beat the original with freshly extracted juice. I would say try *Super Blend Me!* and *Super Juice Me!* on for size when needing a clean up, and see what feels right and works for you. I found that at the end of the 21 days of blends I was craving a freshly extracted juice like crazy, but then juices are a part of my everyday world. If time is an issue but you want a great juice plan, if your budget allows, you can always pop over to www.juicemasterdelivered.com and get one of my plans already made and delivered right to your door!

Q. CAN I DRINK TEA + COFFEE ON THE PLAN?

A. Yes and no. I appreciate that sounds a little vague, but it's my genuine answer! If you want to give the plan 100%, and follow as outlined, then clearly it's a no. However, if a couple of cups of coffee a day is the only way you will stick to it, then it's a yes. There are many extremely good alternatives to coffee and English breakfast tea, such as green and peppermint tea, so why not try these on for size over the first 3 days. Come day 4 – the end of the withdrawal period – chances are you'll be in the herbal tea groove and want to continue.

If you do find yourself at your local coffee house whilst on the plan and still fancy a cheeky caffeine fix, then please heed this advice – **STAY AWAY FROM THE MILKSHAKES POSING AS COFFEES**. Most 'coffees' at these big chains are nothing more than large coffee-flavoured milkshakes. They contain mainly milk, with very little coffee, and if you go for a flavoured option they'll add a generous pump or two of syrup, which will also be loaded with sugar. Herbal teas are definitely the way to go and the good news is, if you order a large one, you can ask for **two** teabags at no extra cost (although it will be hotter than the sun, so ask for ice!). The only downside is, because there's no waiting time, they don't take your name for the cup, so you don't get the chance to make up a random one when asked. Whenever I order a flat white, for example, I'm always Mr. Snuffleupagus (Big Bird's 'imaginary' friend from *Sesame Street*) and I highly recommend, if you do still choose to grab a coffee every now and then, giving the name game a go (or try Engelbert, it works just as well!).

Q. HOW MUCH WEIGHT WILL I LOSE?

A. This depends on a lot of factors. If you are male with weight to lose, chances are you will drop more than a woman with the same amount of weight to lose. This is because men, on average, require more fuel per day than women (due to size, muscle mass and so on). So, when a man and woman with the same weight to lose have the same amount of fuel going in, the man will inevitably drop more weight. If you **don't** have that much weight to lose, then chances are you will only lose what the body wants you to, and then it will regulate itself. If you **do**, then the amount you lose will depend on whether you exercise along with the plan, the type of exercise you do and, of course, whether or not you cheat! The average woman with weight to lose, who does at least 30 minutes of exercise a day alongside the plan, can expect to drop around 5-7lbs by doing the minimum 7-day *Super Blend Me! Challenge*. A man doing the same thing can expect to drop around 7-10lbs. If you do the full 21-day *Super Blend Me! Challenge*, you can expect to drop between 14-20lbs, depending on the factors previously mentioned. There are no hard and fast rules here, and although for many weight loss is one of the main incentives for doing *SBM!*, the overall objective should always be well-being and supplying the body and mind with the right fuel for optimum health – weight loss should never be the *only* focus here.

Q. IS IT SUITABLE FOR VEGANS?

A. Yes. There are some recipes with yoghurt in, but you can use a vegan alternative like coconut yoghurt (as I do).

Q. CAN I EXERCISE ON THE PLAN?

A. Yes, and it's hugely encouraged. This plan has been specifically designed with plenty of plant-based protein, and is therefore ideal for those who wish to exercise at the same time. As I have mentioned a few times throughout the book, I tested *Super Blend Me!* whilst doing high intensity exercise. I actually set myself a 21-day exercise challenge to do alongside the 21-day *Super Blend Me!* plan; to cycle 21 miles a day for 21 days. Clearly I was in the test phase, and doing 21 miles a day at a fast pace, for the duration of the plan, might not be something you fancy doing! However, if you're doing the average *Super Blend Me! Challenge* of 10 days, then I would highly recommend setting yourself a 10-day exercise challenge at the same time. 30 minutes in the morning and 30 minutes in the evening will give good after-burn (see *Rule 5*, page 69, to find out more about this) and won't create too much adrenal fatigue, either. It is up to you, but if you want maximum results then get your body moving a couple of times a day too.

Q. I CAN'T GET HOLD OF A CERTAIN INGREDIENT FOR A RECIPE, WHAT DO I DO?

A. Be smart and just adjust intelligently. For example, if a recipe calls for spinach and kale and you run out kale, just add more spinach. If you can't get hold of cashew butter and can only find almond butter, then just use almond. Run out of coconut milk? Use another milk instead. I think you get the idea – if you can't get hold of one ingredient, simply replace with one which is as close as you can get.

Q. I'M ALLERGIC TO _____ WHAT DO I DO?

A. If you are *genuinely* allergic to any of the ingredients in the recipes, then clearly just leave them out! If you have a nut allergy, then this plan isn't for you – there are just far too many uses of nuts throughout the plan (milk / butter / fresh) to even try to adjust. However, if you're allergic to apples but okay with pears, then just simply swap them out.

Q. HOW MANY CALORIES ROUGHLY PER BLEND?

A. See *Rule 6* (page 71)

Q. I DON'T HAVE A BULLET-TYPE BLENDER; CAN I STILL DO THE PLAN USING ANY BLENDER?

A. Yes, you can do *Super Blend Me!* with any blender. I mention the NutriBullet and NutriBullet Balance in this book because they are very good and the market leaders. I also love the new technology they have come up with, but if you have a different blender, you'll still be good to go. The only thing I would say is that not all blenders are built the same, so just make sure it can do the job. A lot of people tend to buy a new bullet / blender before starting on a plan of this nature, as often, when you invest in something, it gives you an added incentive. It's like when you get some new gym kit, you feel more inspired to work out; in much the same way, a shiny new blender will inspire you to commit to the plan and use it.

Q. I'M DIABETIC, CAN I STILL DO THE PLAN?

A. Yes **and** no! I am not a doctor and I obviously don't know your personal circumstances (like every condition, there's a spectrum of disease) so I'm not really in a position to be able to give you a concrete yes or no. What I will say is that if you have type 2 diabetes, I see no reason on earth why this plan wouldn't be safe for you or even have a positive impact on your condition. Each *Super Blend* has plenty of soluble and insoluble fibre, which acts as a natural buffer against sugar spikes, and most are rich in good fats and protein. There is also the option of two daily *Hunger SOS*s, so in terms of making sure your blood sugars are regulated, we've got it covered. However, as always, I *have to* tell you to *"please consult your doctor first"* (I always find it funny that you don't have to do this before going on a bender in Vegas for a week, but hey!) You know your personal condition far better than I do, so do what feels right for you (*after* you've had a chat with your doctor of course).

Q. I'M FEELING TIRED ON THE PLAN, IS THIS NORMAL?

A. Yes, especially during the first 72 hours, which I refer to as the *withdrawal stage*. However, once you're past that, you should find a good sustained level of energy. It's worth perhaps re-reading *Rule 7* (page 73) as it's also important that you realise that not everything you experience is because of the challenge.

Q. DO I NEED TO DRINK ALL OF MY BLENDS?

A. This varies from person to person, so please see *Rule 3* (page 64)

Q. CAN I FREEZE THE BLENDS?

A. Yes, you can, but why bother? The beauty of *Super Blend Me!* is that you only need your blender. Of all the kitchen appliances, a blender is by far the easiest to clean. A *Super Blend* takes seconds to make, and the blender seconds to clean. Even if you take into account the time it takes to prep the ingredients, the whole process shouldn't take any longer than five minutes. If you have a bullet-type blender, then you can even drink your blend from the cup you made it in – so *even less* washing up. As mentioned, you can freeze your blends, but why bother when it's so quick to blend and enjoy fresh? You are only having three blends a day, so you can make your first two in the morning (take one to work and store in the fridge) and then make your evening *Super Blend* fresh when you get in. Many people, if finances allow, get an extra bullet / blender for the workplace so they can make a fresh blend at lunchtime. Do what works for you, but my advice, if you're going to make them yourself, make them fresh! If you don't fancy making them yourself or shopping for everything, then a version of *Super Blend Me!* can be delivered freshly frozen and delivered direct to your door from *www.juicemasterdelivered.com.*

Q. HOW LONG DO THE BLENDS STAY FRESH?

A. My advice would be to make and drink on the same day (unless freezing).

Q. I WORK NIGHTS SO CAN I ADJUST THE TIME FRAMES ACCORDINGLY?

A. Yes, see *Rule 2* (page 62)

Q. IS IT SUITABLE FOR CHILDREN?

A. Yes **and** no… I think you, as the parent / guardian, need to be the one who makes the decision as to whether it's suitable for *your* child. Kids come in all shapes, ages and sizes and so a blanket yes or no answer simply doesn't fit here. If you have, say, a twelve-year-old who has a genuine weight problem and maybe suffering from various lifestyle conditions, then I'd personally have no issue at all allowing them to do a *Super Blend Me! Challenge.* However, if your kid is in good shape, eats *relatively* well (they're kids, after all, and need to be kids) then I'd say no, don't put them on the plan. The last thing you want to do is to create an issue where perhaps there isn't one. If you are following the plan then sure, make them one or even two a day, but don't have them do the plan if they don't have a *genuine* weight or health issue.

Q. I WANT TO DO TO THE PLAN BUT I DON'T WANT TO LOSE WEIGHT. WHAT DO YOU ADVISE?

A. One the beauties of *Super Blend Me!* is that if you are already lean, you won't wither away on this plan. You have plenty of plant protein and good fats going in and, taking into account the *Hunger SOSs*, at least 1,200 calories a day, so your body will regulate naturally. If you are in good shape already, all that happens is that you end up in *great* shape by the end of the challenge. People who are in pretty good shape and hit the gym love this plan because, in a short space of time, they can get pretty shredded! Clearly, if you don't have any weight to lose, then don't pick the 21-day challenge – dip your toe in for seven days and maybe add an extra blend each day if you feel you need it.

Q. I'M EXTREMELY OVERWEIGHT AND ILL, AM I BETTER OFF DOING YOUR SUPER JUICE ME! PLAN?

A. This completely depends on the individual. If you are someone who is easily put off by the cleaning of the juicer and the extra effort it takes, then the *Super Juice Me!* 28-day plan isn't for you, because you won't *actually* do it. However, if cleaning your juicer isn't an issue, then yes, you are (in my opinion) better off doing the *Super Juice Me!* plan. Whilst I love the simplicity of pure blends, the sheer volume of micronutrients is much greater on a *juice only* plan and therefore if you are really ill and overweight, then it would certainly be the better option. Please don't think, however, that you won't still see significant changes whilst consuming blends, because you will. I just know how stupidly good the results are on *Super Juice Me!* It's your call, but if you do either plan for at least 21 days, you'll be in a different world to the one you are currently in.

Q. I AM ON MEDICATION, SHOULD I CONTINUE WITH IT WHILST ON THE PLAN?

A. Yes, **never** just stop taking your medication. If you start to feel better throughout the course of the challenge then you may wish to talk to your doctor about the possibility of reducing your dosage, but always do this *before* taking action.

Q. CAN I SUBSTITUTE BLENDS IF I DON'T LIKE ONE?

A. Yes, but not from another book or YouTube video! Not because there aren't wonderful recipes out there, but because they may not all fit the *Super Blend Me!* criteria. If you genuinely don't like one of the *Super Blends* (how you can't I don't know, but just imagine) then yes, you can substitute with another blend from the book / app that is similar. For example, if you don't like one of the earthier, green, avocado-based ones, you need to either replace with another green, avocado recipe that you *do* like, or adjust it so you can drink it – (for instance you might try adding in a little more pineapple). The closer you stick to the recipes I have laid out, the better, but I understand not all recipes will be to everyone's taste. If it's just a single ingredient you don't like / can't have, you can simply swap it for something else. If you are replacing avocado, do so with a banana **and** some omega 3,6,9 oil – as you need the good fats! See *Tip 7* (page 89).

Q. WHAT'S THE BEST BLENDER ON THE MARKET FOR THIS PLAN?

A. Please refer to *Rule 3* (page 64).

Q. I'VE FINISHED THE CHALLENGE AND FEEL SO GOOD THAT I DON'T WANT TO STOP. CAN I JUST CARRY ON?

A. Yes. If you still have weight to lose and some health challenges to overcome, there is no reason why you can't continue for a period. However, what I will say is that living on just blends for a very long period of time isn't conducive with normal human existence. So, unless you really feel you *need* to continue, check out the *Life After Super Blend Me!* section of this book (page 219) where you'll find out the best follow-on options available to you. Many people who wish to continue just on blends, tend to go for the *BBM* option, whilst others do the *Super Blend* version of my *2-3-2 System* (don't worry, this will all make sense once you've read the section!) It's up to you, but the *Super Blend Me! Challenge* has been designed as a kick-start, **not** a permanent way of life. I personally do my *2-3-2 System* but mix and match *Super Blends* and juices, depending on my mood and the time I have available.

Q. WHAT SHALL I DO AFTER THE PLAN?

A. Please refer to *Life After Super Blend Me!* section (page 219).

Q. CAN I USE THE BLENDS AS PART OF A 5:2 DIET FOR MAINTENANCE AFTER THE PLAN?

A. Yes. I explain all in *Life After Super Blend Me!* section (page 219).

Q. CAN I USE FROZEN FRUIT AND VEG?

A. Yes. This is the beauty of *Super Blend Me!* You can't *juice* frozen spinach, kale, berries or avocado – but you can *blend* them. Most of the ingredients you'll be using will either be in your cupboard or your freezer, making the plan extremely easy to do and with very little waste. I have added much more weight to this in *Tip 2* of the *7 Tips For Success* (page 77).

Q. PEOPLE AROUND ME ARE TELLING ME IT'S DANGEROUS, SHOULD I LISTEN?

A. No. If you encounter anyone saying anything negative about the fact you're doing this plan, simply tell them to bog off (in the nicest possible way, of course!).

It always astounds me that if you have a week full of junk food and alcohol nobody says a word, but the second you have nothing but good nutrition going into your body for a week, all hell breaks loose. It's dangerous to put your head in an oven, but it's *not* dangerous to do *Super Blend Me!*

Q. AM I BETTER OFF DOING THE PLAN WITH A FRIEND OR FAMILY MEMBER?

A. This depends on your friends and family! If you are doing it with someone, please make sure that you understand that your challenge is personal to you. Your success should not depend or rely on whether the person, or people, you are doing it with stay the course. Although on the surface it may appear you have more chance of success when doing it with someone, at times the opposite can happen. If one person gives in, it can often become their sole objective to make sure the other person gives in too (so *they* don't look like a failure). It's also important not to compare your challenge with anyone else's; whilst the plan is the same, the experience and results will be unique to the individual. Do the challenge with someone by all means, but make sure that if *they* fail they don't drag *you* down with them. This is your challenge and ultimately your success is down to you.

Q. ARE THE SUPPLEMENT POWDERS 100% NECESSARY FOR THE PLAN AND DO I NEED TO GET THE SPECIAL SUPER BLEND ME! POWDERS?

A. Yes **and** no. The protein powder is 100% necessary and an essential part of the plan, but the green and berry powders are completely optional. Having said that, if you want to make the most of your challenge, then I would include them. All of your nutrition is coming from the *Super Blends*, so it's worth making them as nutrient-packed as they can be. As for whether you need to use the **specific** *Super Blend Me!* powders, the answer is no, you don't. I developed the powders to go hand in hand with the plan, but there are many powders on the market to choose from – just do your homework and go for quality. The cheapest is rarely the best, in my experience, and the old saying of *you get what you pay for* is often true when it comes to supplement powders. As protein powder is the only *must have*, it's good to know you can get it almost anywhere. Just avoid things like whey protein if you're vegan. The *Super Blend Me!* protein powder is a combination of pea and hemp, which I feel is the perfect plant-based protein powder. Once again though, it's your choice.

Q. I'M FLYING TODAY, SO WHAT DO I DO AS I CAN'T TAKE LIQUIDS THROUGH CUSTOMS?

A. Firstly, you shouldn't really have picked a time for your challenge when you are flying. I appreciate though, that this isn't always possible, so if you do have to fly here's what to do. You can either replace your blend at the airport for fruit, energy bars or energy balls. Even on a long flight, a few bananas, *good* energy bars or homemade energy balls are usually sufficient. In the recipe section of this book I have some cool energy ball recipes which you can currently take through customs, so even if you're flying you have no excuse. Or, you can simply accept you are flying and that you will need to be more flexible that day. Many just grab a nice salad, which is okay.

Q. CAN I DO IT WHILST BREASTFEEDING OR PREGNANT?

A. Personally I don't see any problem in doing this whether breastfeeding or pregnant but, as always, please consult your doctor first. Once again, it makes me laugh that if someone eats total crap throughout their pregnancy or whilst breastfeeding they don't need to 'consult their doctor' first. It is the mad world we currently live in, so although I'd say yes, you're good to go on both fronts, you need to check with a doctor first, regardless of whether they have studied nutrition or not.

Q. CAN I SMOKE / VAPE?

A. If you are a smoker, I fully understand (as an ex 2-3 packets a day person) that it's not simply a case of saying that you can't smoke on the plan. Nicotine is highly addictive and its invisible pull can be extraordinarily strong. Oh, and if you vape, please be under no illusion that you are free from nicotine addiction – you are as firmly in the trap as any cigarette smoker. Although both smoking and vaping are highly addictive, both can be extremely easy to kick. This sounds like a contradiction, but the addiction to nicotine is around 95% psychological and 5% physical. This means that once you understand how the nicotine trap works, you can release yourself mentally, often even before you've had your last cigarette. It would be impossible for me to explain here as it's a book in itself, so I suggest you download my **100% FREE** *Stop Smoking In 2hrs* app for IOS or Android. You should listen to this *before* you start, so you can be free of cigarettes / vaping throughout *Super Blend Me!* and beyond. You probably had no intention of stopping smoking / vaping when you decided to check out this *Super Blend Me!* thing, but stopping the slavery to nicotine is, without question, the single most important thing you will ever do in your life on the health and freedom front. If you don't want to do the two together (although there is no reason on earth not to, as you'll soon realise once you've listened to the app) then stop nicotine addiction *before* you take on the *Super Blend Me! Challenge*. I saw my beautiful mother suffer the most horrible passing from this world, at the very tender age of just 63, with stage 4 lung cancer, so trust me when I say this will be the last thing you ever want to happen to you. No one wants to go before their time, and don't you want to rree from nicotine's clutches? It is possible, so download this genuinely FREE app (no in-app purchases and all that nonsense) and free yourself now.

Q. HOW MUCH WATER SHOULD I DRINK ON THE CHALLENGE?

A. There are no hard and fast rules here as everyone is different. How much exercise you do will clearly play a huge part in how much water you need to be drinking, but oddly you will find you have less need for water than usual. This is because:

1. You are living on nothing but hydrating liquids, which naturally cuts down the need for more water.

2. You're eliminating foods / drinks, such as alcohol and salt. The best gauge of how much water you should be having is, oddly, thirst (I know, radical!). The blanket piece of advice that says we need two litres of water a day is a total myth, with zero evidence to back it up. When I did the *Super Blend Me! Challenge* I got my hydration through the blends themselves and natural teas. If you are feeling hungry between blends, but not hungry enough to justify a *Hunger SOS*, I found a large cup of green or mint tea did the job. I also love naturally sparkling water with ice and lemon, again a godsend whilst on this plan.

Q. I HAVE ORDERED THE SUPER BLEND ME! PLAN FROM YOUR JUICE DELIVERY COMPANY AND THE CALORIES SEEM LOWER – HOW COME?

A. The bottles over at *Juice Master Delivered* are 420ml but when making the recipes at home, they'll roughly come in at 500ml. To make up the calorie shortfall each delivered plan comes with two Juice SOS energy bars to have each day, in addition to the blends. However, once again, don't get caught up with the numbers – for reasons already mentioned in the book (See *Rule 6* page 71) as I will always have your nutritional back covered. Come the end of your *Super Blend Me!* experience from *Juice Master Delivered*, you'll be feeling and looking so good that any concerns about calories, protein, fats or carbs will have gone out the window!

FIND US ON SOCIAL MEDIA

@juicemaster

facebook.com/juicemasterltd

@jasonvale

youtube.com/juicemaster

GET IN TOUCH

✉

testimonials@juicemaster.com

FIND US ONLINE

www.superblendme.com
www.superjuiceme.com
www.juicemaster.com

FRESH FROZEN JUICE TO YOUR DOOR

www.juicemasterdelivered.com

JUICE MASTER RETREATS

www.juicyoasis.com
www.juicymountain.com

JUICE E-LEARNING

www.juicemasteracademy.com